"A timely and practical book about male sexual function by two highly respected clinicians, this text is of exceptional value because it combines information about biological and psychological treatment in one brief, easily readable text. I would recommend that all men with erectile problems read this book."

> —R. T. Segraves, MD, Ph.D., professor of psychiatry at Case Western School of Medicine and editor of the *Journal of Sex and Marital Therapy*

"Metz and McCarthy have done it again! This time they contribute to our understanding of erectile dysfunction with as much clarity and direction as they did in their earlier volume, *Coping with Premature Ejaculation*. Their new book covers all the bases in guiding the reader to an easy understanding of the assessment, causes, successful treatment, and relapse prevention of a sexual difficulty that has gained so much public and professional attention. *Coping with Erectile Dysfunction* delivers."

> —Julian Slowinski, Psy.D., clinical assistant professor of psychiatry at the University of Pennsylvania School of Medicine, AASECT-certified sex therapist, and coauthor of *The Sexual Male*

"This is a comprehensive book written with professional expertise, confidence, and compassion—a must-read for men and women. Thanks to Metz and McCarthy for making *Coping with Erectile Dysfunction* so informative and hopeful."

> —Pat Love, Ed.D., author of *The Truth About Love*

Coping with Erectile Dysfunction

How to Regain Confidence

& Enjoy Great Sex

MICHAEL E. METZ, PH.D.

BARRY W. MCCARTHY, PH.D.

New Harbinger Publications, Inc.

Publisher's Note

Care has been taken to confirm the accuracy of the information presented and to describe generally accepted practices. However, the authors, editors, and publisher are not responsible for errors or omissions or for any consequences from application of the information in this book and make no warranty, express or implied, with respect to the contents of the publication.

The authors, editors, and publisher have exerted every effort to ensure that any drug selection and dosage set forth in this text are in accordance with current recommendations and practice at the time of publication. However, in view of ongoing research, changes in government regulations, and the constant flow of information relating to drug therapy and drug reactions, the reader is urged to check the package insert for each drug for any change in indications and dosage and for added warnings and precautions. This is particularly important when the recommended agent is a new or infrequently employed drug.

Some drugs and medical devices presented in this publication may have Food and Drug Administration (FDA) clearance for limited use in restricted research settings. It is the responsibility of the health care provider to ascertain the FDA status of each drug or device planned for use in their clinical practice.

Distributed in Canada by Raincoast Books.

Copyright © 2004 by Michael Metz and Barry McCarthy
New Harbinger Publications, Inc.
5674 Shattuck Avenue
Oakland, CA 94609

Cover design by Amy Shoup
Cover image by PhotoAlto/Picturequest
Text design by Michele Waters-Kermes

ISBN 1-57224-386-4 Paperback

Printed in the United States of America

New Harbinger Publications' Web site address: www.newharbinger.com

06   05   04

10   9   8   7   6   5   4   3   2   1

First printing

Contents

Dedication and Acknowledgments

I gratefully dedicate this book to my wife, Hildy Bowbeer, who has always encouraged my work, and thank her for our years of sharing life and family. I also want to thank Harold Lief, MD, a central influence during my training and then practice in sexual therapy for many years; and Norman Epstein, Ph.D., a major leader in cognitive behavioral therapy with couples, who has substantially influenced my work for many years as a teacher, colleague, and friend.

—M.E.M.

I dedicate this book to my two grandchildren, Torren Michael McCarthy and Daphne Jeannette McCarthy, with the hope that they grow up in a world where healthy sexuality is valued and sexual dysfunction, including ED, is much less prevalent.

—B.W.M.

This book represents what we have learned from the several thousand people we have clinically treated, and from the scientific research and clinical experience of our sex therapy colleagues. Many of these are associates in the Society for Sex Therapy and Research (SSTAR), the American Association of Sex Education, Counseling and Therapy (AASECT), the Society for the Scientific Study of Sexuality (SSSS), the Association for Advancement of Behavioral Therapy (AABT), the American Association for Marital and Family Therapy (AAMFT), and the American Psychological Association (APA).

We also want to acknowledge the outstanding contributions of the people we have happily worked with at New Harbinger Publications: Spencer Smith, acquisitions editor;   Jessica Beebe, copy editor; Amy Shoup, art director;   Gretchen Gold, web manager, permissions, and advertising;   Troy DuFrene, marketing and sales;   Michele Waters, director of production; and Heather Mitchener, editorial director. Thank you all.

—Michael E. Metz
Barry W. McCarthy

Introduction

Erectile dysfunction (ED), defined as a problem with getting or keeping an erection sufficient for intercourse, is very common. Most men experience this sexual difficulty periodically, but when erections are consistently unpredictable, ED becomes a personal and relationship crisis. For a man and his partner who enjoyed satisfying sex before having ED, this experience can be intensely disturbing, creating anxiety, self-blame, and relationship stress. There is an increasing amount of data demonstrating that by age fifty, approximately 50 percent of men complain about their erectile functioning and feel they have ED, at least in its mild form (Feldman et al. 1994). That is a very sobering statistic.

ED AND VIAGRA

In the 1950s, most professionals believed that ED was caused by childhood psychological problems. Masters and Johnson (1970) revolutionized research in human sexual behavior by demonstrating that "performance anxiety" was a major cause of ED. But in 1998, the medical and public approach to understanding and treating ED shifted dramatically with the introduction of Viagra (sildenafil). Now the pendulum has swung to the opposite belief; it is popularly believed that almost all ED is caused by physiological factors, especially vascular problems, rather than psychological issues or relationship distress.

In television ads for Viagra, former senator and presidential candidate Bob Dole was a very persuasive spokesman, identifying ED as a medical problem requiring a medical treatment. The message he delivered was this: All a man with ED need do is talk to his doctor and get a Viagra prescription. In later ads, a woman was given the supportive role of encouraging the man to ask his doctor if Viagra was right for him. The message, although simplistic, was beneficial: ED is not your fault; speak out and get help. However, the second, subtle part of the message was not helpful: ED has a single (medical) cause and a simple cure (Viagra).

The Viagra revolution was certainly valuable in that it challenged the silence and stigma regarding ED. We should never return to the secrecy and shame of the past. Now, the media and medical professionals regularly advocate the "magic blue pill"—and newer versions such as Levitra (vardenafil) and Cialis (tadalafil). However, this medical approach to ED oversimplifies the problem and promises more than it can deliver. ED is more complex than such a simple problem–simple cure promise. Although the achievement of an erection is very important, a healthy, fulfilling sexual relationship is much more intricate than such a mechanistic view allows. This truth becomes evident when you realize that for every man who has been helped by Viagra, an equal number—and perhaps many more—have "failed" with Viagra. Such men (and couples) may feel even more stigmatized and sexually demoralized after trying Viagra and not succeeding than before using Viagra.

IS THIS BOOK FOR YOU?

The goals of our book are to present an honest picture of male sexuality, to describe what ED is and is not, to offer suggestions on how to approach and change the problem of ED, and to present a comprehensive, *biopsychosocial* (biological, psychological, and social) approach that involves both you and your partner. This new approach to male and couple sexuality offers realistic hope and a workable plan to enhance sexual desire, pleasure, and satisfaction. The essence of our approach is that the man has to assume responsibility for adopting a new model for sexual pleasure and arousal, while the couple works together to rebuild comfort and confidence with erections.

If you've picked up this book hoping for a quick and easy cure that guarantees effortless and predictable erections 100 percent of the time, you've picked up the wrong book. Too many men and their partners have become disillusioned with the quick and easy approach, including the new myth that ED can be cured with a pill alone. That approach entirely misses the point that sexuality is a complex experience shared by a couple.

In this book, we'll present an honest, scientifically valid, clinically relevant approach that can help the great majority of men develop a functional and satisfying sexual relationship. Ideally, this will not only change your present ED problem but will also help you learn new healthy attitudes, behaviors, and feelings that will inoculate you against sexual problems in the future.

I

Understanding Erectile Dysfunction: Myths and Realities

Before we present our biopsychosocial approach for understanding and changing erectile dysfunction, let's first see what you and your partner know about sex and ED. Take the following true-false test individually, and then compare your answers.

Few young men have an unsuccessful first intercourse experience, but if they do, this signals they will have a lifelong sexual problem.	True	False
Only 5 percent of all men experience an erection problem before age forty.	True	False
Smoking does not affect sexual functioning.	True	False
If the woman does not perform like the man (that is, have one orgasm during intercourse with no additional stimulation), it means he is an inadequate lover.	True	False
The larger the man's penis in the flaccid state, the larger it is in the erect state. Penis size is the best measure of virility.	True	False
Simultaneous orgasm is the best goal for couples to aspire to, and this requires a very hard erection.	True	False
Successful intercourse is totally the man's responsibility, and intercourse failure is totally his fault.	True	False
A real man can have an erection with any woman, any time, in any situation.	True	False
The major cause of ED is low testosterone.	True	False

For most men, penile injections are more comfortable than taking Viagra.	True	False
Prostate surgery is to be avoided at all costs because it invariably results in impotence.	True	False
ED is usually the woman's fault.	True	False
Viagra results in firm erections 100 percent of the time.	True	False
Less than 10 percent of men drop out of Viagra treatment.	True	False
A normal consequence of aging is the loss of capacity to have an erection.	True	False

How many of the above statements did you mark true? In fact, they are all false. This test is composed entirely of sexual myths. The average man believes six of these myths to be true. For health professionals, the average number believed true is three. Old myths grew from lack of information and repressive attitudes; new myths arise from commercial exaggeration and unrealistic performance demands.

Myths die hard. These myths subvert male sexuality and set you up to fail at overcoming ED. Male sex myths are based on a competitive model of what it means to be a man, especially a sexual man. Asking questions or admitting weaknesses is not part of the traditional male role. So it is not "cool" or "masculine" to challenge a myth or admit that you don't know something, are unsure, or have "failed." Perhaps one man in four has an unsuccessful first intercourse experience, usually because he ejaculates before beginning intercourse, loses an erection, or can't get a condom on right. However, rather than admit the difficulty, he tells his friends the woman thought he was the best ever and begged him to come back to have sex again. This bravado can be funny, but it reinforces a competitive, performance-oriented, isolated, and basically fear-based approach to male sexuality. You always have to prove yourself sexually, both to the woman and to your male friends. Your partner is not your sexual friend. She is someone to perform for, and you fear that if you fail, she will judge you as not man enough and tell other people you are a sexual loser.

Knowledge is power. The more clearly you and your partner understand the physical, psychological, relational, and sexual technique factors that contribute to healthy sexuality, the better. The most important concept to understand and accept is that sexuality, especially erectile functioning, is complex, not simple.

■ Drew and Melissa

Drew could not believe that he was "impotent" at the age of thirty-two. He recalled with relish his first sexual intercourse at sixteen, an active sex life throughout college and law school, and great sex with Melissa when he was twenty-four and she twenty-five. How could it be that eight years later he was trapped in a nonsexual marriage?

Melissa was very interested in revitalizing their sexual relationship, which had been troubled for the past four years with frequent bouts of ED. For the last two years, Drew had completely stopped trying to be sexual. What had gone wrong? Was it her fault? His? The stress of two careers and two children? Does marriage kill sexual desire? And, most important, was there anything Drew could do to overcome ED and revitalize their sexuality?

Several months earlier, Drew had visited a medical sex clinic that advertised on sports radio. First he tried Viagra, and he did get an erection but lost it during intercourse. He didn't tell Melissa that he was using Viagra. She was very encouraging about trying again, but Drew felt discouraged. He wanted to have erections like the ones he remembered from his teens and twenties: easy, automatic, and predictable. He wanted an "erection to show," not an "erection to grow."

The doctor at the clinic did not ask Drew any psychological or relationship questions; instead, he recommended a more powerful medical intervention, Caverject (alprostadil). The doctor explained that Drew would inject the medication directly into the penis, resulting in increased blood flow and a firm erection. He showed Drew how to do Caverject injections, which did result in a rock-hard erection.

Although Drew felt awkward injecting himself at home and experienced some discomfort with the injection, it did deliver as promised. Again, Drew hid the fact that he was using a medical intervention from Melissa. She seemed quite pleased with two quick, successful intercourses. However, the third time, Melissa asked him to slow down and touch her. When she reached out to stroke his penis, Drew reflexively turned away, which created an awkward feeling between them. Drew's desire and feeling of arousal disappeared, but the erection didn't. What do you do with a firm erection when both people are obviously turned off? Melissa pressed Drew about what happened, but he felt embarrassed and defensive, and wouldn't talk about it. She eventually gave up trying to talk about the experience. Their sex life came to a standstill.

For several months, Drew's sexual outlet was masturbating to computer images and then to visually interactive cybersex. This culminated in a monthly credit card bill of over $400 in charges for computer sex. Drew had prided himself on being a rational problem solver and a fiscal conservative. Clearly, his problem with ED was causing him to act in ways that were both embarrassing and self-defeating.

Finally, Drew talked to his family practitioner, Dr. Lange, about treatment for ED. The physician had known Drew, Melissa, and their children for almost seven years. Melissa had spoken to Dr. Lange about Drew's ED and sexual avoidance three years ago. He'd told her that he would be glad to write a prescription for Viagra but Drew had never asked.

When Drew described his experiences with Viagra and Caverject (he was too embarrassed to disclose his experiences with cybersex), Dr. Lange said that he would be glad to prescribe one of the new generation of ED drugs, Cialis. He also wisely advised Drew to approach the ED problem with Melissa's help and recommended a sex therapist who worked with couples. However, Drew wanted to see whether he and Melissa could overcome the ED on their own with just the help of Cialis. Drew agreed to schedule a follow-up consultation in three months to discuss his sexual progress.

This time Drew told Melissa that he was taking Cialis. He also told her that he needed her help to regain comfort and self-confidence both with his erections and with having intercourse. Dr. Lange had told him that Cialis allows more freedom for initiating sexual relations because it provides a wider window of opportunity (up to thirty-six hours). This helped Drew feel less self-conscious. Its benefit for Melissa was the feeling of a genuine sexual coming together. She knew that Drew was responding to her, not to a pill.

Melissa was very open to helping. She wanted Drew to really try, not to shut down at the first sign of a problem. Melissa told Drew that it was important to her to keep an intimate connection. With enthusiasm for restarting their sexual relationship, Cialis, and Melissa's active involvement, they had three successful intercourse experiences. However, the fourth time, Drew's erection weakened just as he was ready to insert his penis into her vagina. Although Melissa wanted them to continue pleasuring each other and try intercourse later, Drew felt frustrated and demoralized, and turned away.

Melissa was not willing to allow another long stretch of time to go by without having sexual relations. She insisted they go together for a "coaching" session with their physician. Dr. Lange told them that as a rule, family doctors are not used to seeing couples together, especially for sexual concerns, but that he would do his best to help them. He did keep up with the latest scientific findings, and he assured Drew and Melissa that it was typical among success-ful users of Viagra and Cialis for 65 to 80 percent of their attempts, rather than the desired 100 percent, to result in successful intercourse. In fact, what Drew experienced was in the normal range. Dr. Lange recommended that Drew change his expectations, not his medication.

The concept of a variable sexual response was easier for Melissa to accept than it was for Drew. He would have preferred a medication that could guarantee erection and intercourse. Melissa said she enjoyed erotic, nonintercourse sex and so could Drew. She did not have to say it, but Drew was aware that even in the best of their sexual times, Melissa was not orgas-mic every time. He also knew that she still appreciated and enjoyed the touch-ing and intimacy.

Nothing succeeds like success, and in well over 85 percent of their sexual encounters both Drew and Melissa enjoyed themselves. A major breakthrough occurred when Drew lost his erection and rather than backing away, he fol-lowed Melissa's request for manual stimulation. She was orgasmic, and then she stimulated him to erection and put him inside. This was a highly erotic, satisfying experience. The next day, while on a walk, they discussed that encounter, and Melissa made the point that she did not need an erect penis for sexual satisfaction, but she did want an involved Drew.

When Drew was not distracted with monitoring his erection, sex became more fun for both of them. Drew realized he was more emotionally open and sexually free when he was the giving partner, but when he was receiving, he became more tentative and less responsive. Drew told Melissa that he became especially self-conscious when he was passive during sex. He preferred mutual give-and-take pleasuring rather than taking turns. The combination of Melissa's sexual responsivity, Drew's enjoyment of mutual stimulation, the use of Cialis, having realistic expectations, and greater openness to erotic, nonintercourse scenarios greatly improved their marital sexuality.

Drew began to wonder whether he should use Cialis each time. Melissa wanted him to feel responsible for his desire and arousal, and left the decision to him. She felt that with their enhanced intimacy and eroticism, consistent use of Cialis might be unnecessary. Eventually, Drew decided to phase out the medication, but he decided that he would use it again if he had trouble keeping an erection during three encounters in a row. He did not want to reinstate per-formance anxiety. Melissa came up with a plan, too. Her plan called for them to have a fun, erotic date once a month. To encourage sexual playfulness and improvisation, this monthly date would prohibit intercourse entirely.

Drew and Melissa's experience examines the detrimental effects of ED and illustrates the kind of cooperation required of a couple to overcome it. Our biopsychosocial model will help you understand, assess, and overcome your ED.

WHAT IS ED?

Do medical and sexual health professionals agree on an objective definition of ED? Not really. The traditional definitions focused on the percentage of intercourse failures. Masters and Johnson (1970) defined ED as failing at intercourse more than 25 percent of the time. But what if you have unsuccessful intercourse (that is, fail to maintain a sufficiently strong erection for *intromission*—insertion of the penis into the vagina—and intravaginal ejaculation) only 15 percent of the time, but when it occurs you feel a devastating sense of personal and sexual failure? Or what if you have strong erections, but you ejaculate and lose your erection before your penis enters her vagina? Or suppose you have good erections with oral sex or during masturbation, but not during intercourse? Or what if intercourse takes place for more than twenty minutes, but you experience *ejaculatory inhibition* and cannot come? Many men with ejaculatory inhibition eventually lose their erection and misdiagnose themselves as having ED.

If you seldom get an erection or you avoid trying to have sex because of fear, clearly you are suffering from ED. On the other hand, if you are usually successful with intercourse but sometimes fail—whether once every ten times, once a month, or once a year—this is well within the range of normal sexual response and is not considered ED. A comprehensive definition of ED centers on a lack of comfort and confidence with erection, which can involve a variety of contributing factors.

ED IS A BIOPSYCHOSOCIAL PHENOMENON

As in other areas of health and mental health, professionals debate the physical versus the psychological causes of ED. For a number of years, the view was that most cases of ED were psychological in origin, while more recently the approach has been that most cases were physical in their origin. Such either-or views are incomplete and obscure the fact that any important human difficulty has many causes, dimensions, and effects. We invite you to adopt the idea that *ED is a biopsychosocial phenomenon with physical, cognitive, behavioral, and emotional features, as well as identity, cooperation, and emotional intimacy relationship features.* Attending to all of these factors will improve your understanding and assessment of ED and increase the effectiveness of your plan for change. The old saying, "If your only tool is a hammer, every problem looks like a nail," is a clever reminder of the need for a comprehensive view.

Physiological Factors

Anything that subverts your health—poor health habits, untreated medical problems, or side effects of medication—ultimately will subvert your sexual response and erections.

Health Habits

Your eating, exercise, and sleep patterns can contribute to ED. There is increasing evidence that smoking has a long-term negative impact on sexual health because it causes respiratory and vascular deterioration, and alcohol and drug abuse have been shown to subvert sexual function and contribute to ED (Cocones and Gold 1989). Many men use alcohol to lower inhibitions and self-consciousness. Alcohol is a central nervous system depressant; it physiologically inhibits sexual response. In youth, the psychological effects of two or more drinks usually overcame the negative physiological effects. Some men learn to be sexual while high or drunk, but as they age, the physiological effects become stronger, resulting in ED. The man may discover that when he tries to be sexual without using alcohol, he feels like an awkward, self-conscious fourteen-year-old. This is a common complaint of men in Alcoholics Anonymous and a frequent reason for an alcoholic relapse. Taking control of your sexual health means confronting unhealthy habits such as smoking, alcohol and drug abuse, weight gain, lack of exercise, and inadequate sleep.

Vascular, Neurological, and Hormonal Health

Physiologically, there are three systems that affect erections: vascular, neurological, and hormonal. An underlying medical problem in one of these three systems can cause or contribute to ED. Often, ED and other sexual problems are the side effects of certain medications, especially those used to treat high blood pressure and depression. Occasionally, ED is the first symptom of a major medical problem.

In some ways the physical assessment is the easiest. The major question is whether you can obtain firm erections by any means: waking erections, masturbatory erections, erections with manual or oral sex, or erections using idiosyncratic stimuli like a fetish or cybersex. If you can, the likelihood is that your hormonal, vascular, and neurological systems are functional and there is no need for further physical assessment. If you can't, or if you have concerns about your physiological functioning, we suggest you begin by consulting with your family physician. He or she will review your health history and determine whether you have an underlying health problem such as diabetes, high blood pressure, or a neurological disorder. Your physician may refer you to a urologist or sexual medicine specialist for other diagnostic tests.

In addressing concerns about vascular, neurological, and hormonal problems, you need to be an active, aware health advocate for yourself. This means talking to your physician about your concerns, being able to describe your symptoms, and following through with appropriate diagnostic tests. If a medical problem is found, you need to be a knowledgeable and active patient. Develop a communicative relationship with your physician so that you can discuss your concerns openly.

Your Partner's Health

It is also advisable for your partner to assess her general and sexual health status, especially if she is experiencing a sexual dysfunction. Her sexual difficulties, anxieties, and inhibitions can add to your ED and subvert the change process.

Maintaining Factors

Health factors can cause ED, but just treating the health problem or improving your health habits may not be enough to restore your confidence with erections. In other words, what originally caused ED may or may not be what is maintaining it. The experience of ED itself can create psychological and relational distress. For example, it is quite common that couples undergoing infertility treatment develop inhibited sexual desire and ED. Even after they successfully have a baby, a significant number of couples report the stress of the experience resulted in continued psychological, relational, and sexual problems, including ED (Zoldbrod 1993).

Psychological Factors

Psychological factors are particularly important because they can affect not only erections but also sexual desire. These factors can include general psychological stress as well as thoughts or fears specifically about ED.

Any negative emotion—especially anxiety, depression, obsessiveness, or anger—can subvert erectile function. Anxiety about money, sadness over death of a parent or friend, concern about your adolescent child, or loss of a job can interfere with erectile response.

Anticipatory anxiety about ED and other mental distractions about sexual performance are sexual poisons. You want to reinforce the cycle of positive anticipation, pleasure-oriented sexual experiences, and a regular rhythm of sexual contact instead of falling into a pattern of anticipatory anxiety, tense and failed sexual performance, and embarrassment and avoidance. When you view intercourse as a pass-fail test, you are constantly afraid that you are one failure away from feeling totally impotent. We use the term "erectile dysfunction" because it describes the problem for what it is: difficulty with getting and maintaining an erection sufficient for intercourse. "Impotence" connotes a lack of personal power or self-esteem as a man. ED is a problem with your penis going up and down, not a problem with your whole life or with your adequacy as a man.

ED provides an excellent example of how the desire for the perfect cure can subvert the change process. Perfectionism is the enemy of good-enough sexuality. We believe that any man can overcome his embarrassment and denial and address ED both hopefully and realistically. The positive, realistic expectation we suggest you cultivate is that 85 percent of your sexual encounters will flow into intercourse. For the 15 percent of sexual encounters that do not involve intercourse, you and your partner can make a comfortable transition to a nonintercourse backup scenario that is erotic or sensual.

Relationship Factors

Relationship factors—especially comfort, attraction, trust, and intimate cooperation—can facilitate sexual response and erections. Conversely, relationship problems—especially emotional conflict, not feeling close or safe, disappointment with your spouse or marriage, lack of couple time, guilt, or blaming—will undermine the interpersonal connection you need for erectile confidence.

A serious flaw in the medical approach to ED is that it focuses solely on the man. Seldom is he even asked about his relationship. But sexuality is not an individual, isolated event. It is an interpersonal process. ED is best understood and treated using a couple approach. Think for a moment: Sex is not just for you, nor is it just for her. Sex is for you as a couple. Your ED is also her ED. In addressing ED, your partner has an active role to play.

The challenge for couples dealing with ED is to establish a mutually comfortable level of intimacy, one that invites sexual desire and eroticism. Being a cooperative, intimate sexual team is your optimal strategy. There are two extreme modes of behavior to avoid. One is enmeshment (giving up your individuality), where you become so close that there is no space for sexuality. The other is settling into anger, blaming, and alienation.

Your Partner's Response to ED

Many women respond to ED in one of two extreme ways, both of which exacerbate the problem. The most common response is to be "motherly" or conciliatory, saying intimacy is what counts, not sex. In her efforts to be helpful, she may instead send her partner an antierotic message. The other extreme response is for the woman to become sexually demanding, saying that her partner owes her intercourse, and if he can't succeed at intercourse, as compensation he should service her and make sure she has an orgasm. There is nothing intimate, loving, or inviting in that approach.

The healthiest role is for the woman to be a caring, involved sexual friend. If you both feel sexually self-conscious and tentative, this builds an anxious, antierotic atmosphere that compounds your ED. It is helpful if your partner maintains her desire and arousal, because this invites your desire and arousal. However, your partner may not respond in such a positive manner. She may feel hurt or confused when you do not have an easy erection. Some women feel at fault or inadequate, believing they are not sexy enough or not doing the right thing; others feel ED is a rejection and react with anger.

Psychosexual Skill Factors

Psychosexual skill factors involve cognitive, behavioral, emotional, and relationship skills. As your relationship ages and you pass age thirty, psychosexual skills play an increasingly important role. In truth, almost all men say they preferred it when they had guaranteed erections, were not self-conscious about managing the sequence of foreplay, and would proceed to intercourse on their first erection. This scenario is vulnerable in two major ways. First, this is an unrealistic expectation for most men over thirty, the great majority of men over forty, and almost all men over fifty. Second, once you have been sensitized to an erection problem, you simply cannot pretend you are sure of guaranteed, autonomous erections. This does not mean that all men will have ED. It does mean that you need to be open to nonintercourse sexual scenarios and to cognitive, behavioral, and emotional techniques that facilitate arousal and erection.

Situational Factors

Situational factors include issues of private places to be sexual, times to be sexual, and external and emotional factors which subvert sexual function. You may be unaware of the barriers that are in the way. For example, trying to be sexual after midnight when you are exhausted can subvert sexual response. Sex may seem less inviting if you fear that your children are going to barge into the room. Couples find a lock on their bedroom door is of more value than a $20,000 house remodeling. You need to feel secure in order to be sexually responsive.

Some men discover doing little things—being the primary parent for two nights in a row, putting the toilet seat down, talking with your spouse for ten minutes while cleaning the kitchen together, calling just to talk rather than to arrange logistics—can establish a positive couple tone. Consider what practical and situational factors invite a sexual encounter. Equally important, identify the practical and situational factors that subvert a sexual encounter and raise the likelihood of ED.

UNDERSTANDING TREATMENT ISSUES

The idea of a simple approach to "curing" ED (using pills, vitamins, or creams) is growing in popularity, especially in the media and advertising worlds. Men like the idea of a simple, guaranteed solution for ED. Who wouldn't wish for something that ends the problem forever? This is understandable, especially when you're flooded with commercial marketing. Advertisers know that if you are told there is a simple solution, you are more apt to buy the product.

Most men would rather get help from a physician than have to involve their partner in solving the problem of ED. Realize that this disenfranchises her from the very important sexual component of relationship intimacy. This approach is self-defeating. Keep in mind that if you only take a pill, you gain no skill. Even if you have a simple physical cause for ED, be mindful that this problem—even though it can be corrected with medication—exists in the context of your relationship. Satisfying sex is the result of living as an intimate team.

Incorporating Medication

Medical interventions such as Viagra, Levitra, or Cialis can be a vital resource in treatment. The challenge is to integrate the drug into your couple sexual style that involves intimacy, pleasuring, and eroticism. Do not try to use a medication as a stand-alone intervention to give you perfect, 100 percent predictable erections. If you do so, you will likely feel disappointed and demoralized, and you may fall into the trap of a nonsexual relationship. Use all your resources, but use them wisely.

In planning a change program, we suggest a "both-and" approach. Reading this book, talking with your partner, engaging in assessment and behavior change exercises, changing erectile and relationship expectations, and building feelings of intimacy and cooperation will facilitate erectile comfort and confidence. But so can seeing a physician and using medication (for example, testosterone, Cialis, Viagra, Levitra, or an antianxiety medication). If ED does not easily change, this does not mean you are a failure. It is a sign of wisdom to seek and utilize all the resources available to you to overcome your ED. Consulting a couple sex therapist is one of the best decisions and best resources.

Making an Individualized Plan

The key is to understand the causes and effects of your ED, approach ED with a change plan using all needed interventions, work with your partner as an intimate ally, and maintain motivation and focus. This is not a competition between self-help, medical help, and psychotherapy, but an integrated, comprehensive approach to success-fully resolve your ED. To overcome your ED, you must understand and address it with an individualized approach, a plan that fits you and your distinct situation.

Preventing Relapse

The goal is not for you to have ever-ready erections or to prove to yourself or anyone else that you can do it. The goal is to establish comfort and confidence with erections so that you and your partner can again enjoy a satisfying sexual relationship. You don't want to set yourself up for failure by doing well for a month or a year, only to relapse. You can't treat sex with benign neglect; you need to continue to put time and energy into maintaining a healthy sexuality. This includes developing expectations about erectile function that are both positive and realistic.

2

A New Integrative Model of Male Sexuality

The essence of ED is that you have lost your comfort and confidence with erections and intercourse. ED is a changeable problem. The goal of ED treatment is not just to restore erections and resume intercourse but to establish a new way of understanding desire, pleasure, arousal, intercourse, and couple sexuality that will allow you to maintain your gains and help prevent further problems with ED as you and your relationship age. Increasing sexual awareness and adopting positive, realistic sexual expectations is part of a new, healthy model of male sexuality.

You do not need to be the sexual Lone Ranger or take the Superman approach to sex and erections. At core, sexuality is an interpersonal process. Overcoming ED is a couple challenge, not solely your burden. The new model of male sexuality focuses broadly on intimacy and shared pleasure rather than narrowly on intercourse performance. Intimate, interactive sex is more satisfying than autonomous, performance-oriented sex.

Our approach to sexuality is biopsychosocial in that it addresses the physical, psychological, relational, and situational aspects of sexuality and ED and teaches you psychosexual skills. This new model of male sexuality is integrative in that it recognizes that dichotomous (either-or) thinking is limited. Including all the dimensions and using all your resources offers the best plan for success and genuine growth.

ADULT SEXUALITY IS A LIFELONG PROCESS

Recent studies that compared the quality of sex of singles, cohabiting couples, and married couples found that the best quality sex is in marriage

(Michael et al. 1994). But how can this be? Marital sex is supposed to be routine, boring, lethargic, and perfunctory. In fact, married couples enjoy stable sex with benefits like comfort, relaxation, trust, pleasure, cooperation, and emotional intimacy. Satisfying marital sex is respectful, tender, playful, occasionally experimental, and integrated into real life amidst careers, kids, and routines. Healthy sexuality is honest and realistic; it fits your lifestyle as well as at times providing an escape.

Youthful Sex Is Automatic

The typical young man is very sexually confident and unselfconscious. Erections are spontaneous, easy, highly predictable, and automatic. Most important, erections are autonomous—you don't need stimulation from your partner. Masculine self-esteem and sexuality are closely associated. Because adolescents and young adults consider sexuality to be such a simple matter, it is hard to convince adult men to think differently about sexuality. There are a number of sexual issues that young men do worry about: an unwanted pregnancy, sexually transmitted diseases and HIV, penis size, premature ejaculation, and whether they're having as much sex as their peers. However, young men usually do not worry about sexual desire or erections.

Beer commercials, movies, and "reality" TV reinforce the idea that male sexuality is youthful, illicit, wild and easy, and requires no intimacy, cooperation, or mutual pleasuring. In R-rated films, sex is always short, intense, nonverbal, perfect, and—most important—the man is always turned on before they even begin. Interestingly, marital sex is rarely portrayed in movies; more often, it is premarital sex or an extramarital affair. Porn videos present an even more unrealistic model. The porn star always has a firm erection no matter what, and the theme is that the crazier the woman and the more bizarre the situation, the more erotic it is. This is an insane model of sexuality.

Mature Sex Is Interpersonal

Eventually, the easy, automatic sexual functioning of youth begins to change. Some of the reason for change is physiological; your hormonal, vascular, and neurological systems are most efficient from ages sixteen to twenty-two. That is when you are at your peak as a sexual athlete, which is quite different than being an intimate lover. Some men think that they need to have all the sex they can in their twenties because it's all downhill after that. What a limited, self-defeating way to understand the role and meaning of sexuality. Sexuality is neither an athletic event nor a performance competition but a pleasure-oriented, meaningful human experience. At its best, sexuality integrates pleasuring and eroticism, mutual acceptance, emotional intimacy, and spiritual union. It serves as an important part of the "emotional glue" of your relationship. You don't have to wait until your forties to learn this. Even in your twenties, you can enjoy and value intimate sexuality.

As you age, your relationships become more important and mature. Until this growth occurs, it is common for men to go to one of two extremes, either ignoring the woman's sexual feelings or taking on the job of being sure she has an orgasm during intercourse every time. Her orgasm becomes the measure of your sexual performance. In a healthy relationship, you view the woman as your partner in sharing feelings, pleasure, and eroticism.

In a serious relationship, sex expands to include the many ways you use your bodies for closeness, affection, soothing, consoling, pleasing, playfulness, and excitement. Sharing your lives provides the opportunity to experience your sexual interactions in a subtly yet distinctively personalized and enriched way: sex on vacation, during pregnancy, during times of loneliness, after the wedding of your best friend, after a parent's death, during times of career stress, after a class reunion, during periods of success and achievement, in times of illness, during unemployment, during childrearing, after business travel or a long absence such as military service, after conflict with your teenager, during your adjustment to the "empty nest," adapting to changes with aging, during retirement. Who you are and what you are living through during each stage of your life can personalize your sexual experiences. One time, sex is for anxiety release through orgasm, another time for escape and fun, another time for emotional healing, another time as a spiritual experience such as having gentle intercourse while you share your sadness about your dad's death a month earlier. Younger couples are frequently surprised that real couples have such a variety of sexual experiences and meanings.

The new model of male sexuality encourages you to approach sexuality as a lifelong developmental process, a vital aspect of your personality ripe for new learning, personal growth, and enhanced intimacy whatever your age. The youthful biological urge for procreation and physical pleasure can develop into wise self-esteem and emotional intimacy that deepens as you integrate sexuality into your lives and relationship. This healthier model of male sexuality will help you overcome ED and learn to have sex that is not only physically pleasurable but also emotionally intimate. This will help you avoid sexual problems associated with your aging and the aging of your relationship, and help you handle the vicissitudes of your lives.

PERSONAL RESPONSIBILITY

The new model of male sexuality involves personal responsibility. This means that each person is responsible for his or her own desire, arousal, and orgasm. You are no longer responsible for the woman sexually; the entire burden is not on you. Sex is a shared activity, not a pass-fail test where you feel responsible for any experience that is not perfect.

VARIABLE, FLEXIBLE SEXUALITY

This new model defines a sexual connection more broadly than intercourse. Does a sensual, playful, or erotic encounter count if it does not result in intercourse? The traditional view was that the only real sex is intercourse. The new view of a variable, flexible couple sexuality is that oral sex, manual sex, playful genital touching, and nongenital pleasuring can all offer a meaningful couple connection. If you do not have an erection sufficient for intercourse, it is okay to change the scenario to erotic, nonintercourse sex (oral or manual pleasuring, for example) or a close, sensual experience that ends the encounter positively.

Can you feel good about nonintercourse scenarios, or do you experience this as a sexual failure? Men commonly believe they cannot develop this flexibility, feeling they'll "die of blue balls" (frustration) if they choose to forgo ejaculation now and then. It is not easy, and it requires strength and self-regulation, but it is a liberating aspect of couple sexuality. It removes performance anxiety for both of you. Couples who adopt a broader, more flexible approach to sexuality will have a resilient and satisfying sexual life.

BEING AN INTIMATE TEAM

Perhaps the most important factor in the new model of male sexuality is viewing the woman as your intimate friend. To work as an intimate team will require changes not only for you but for your partner as well. She may be in the habit of expecting you to initiate sexual encounters with a spontaneous, autonomous erection. The wise and open woman accepts and embraces the opportunity to develop an intimate, interactive sexual relationship. Arousal can be a synergistic process in which each person's sexual responsiveness invites and enhances the other's arousal. You can learn to piggyback your arousal on her arousal. It helps to know that for most couples, with aging, female arousal is easier and more predictable than male arousal. Her desire is good for you and your relationship. A sexually excited partner is the best aphrodisiac. The man who welcomes, enjoys, and responds to his partner's arousal has a major sexual resource.

Few women have absolutely predictable arousal and orgasm. Even the most sexually responsive woman experiences a fluctuating sexual response pattern. She likely accepts a variable sexual response for herself, and can learn to accept this for you. Can you accept this for yourself? Can you embrace and enjoy a new model of male sexuality in which desire and arousal are a function of your emotional and erotic interaction?

DEVELOPING HEALTHY SEXUAL SCENARIOS

Developing a shared understanding of sex as cooperative, intimate, and erotic is very important in addressing your ED. Sexual scenarios are the "movies" in your mind about what the sexual experience can be like. Scenarios learned early in life often subvert male sexuality in adulthood because when young men think of foreplay, they invariably think of the man stimulating the woman to get her ready for intercourse. In this scenario, sex is a one-way highway leading to the destination of intercourse.

By the time within a sexual encounter when most men feel open to receiving the woman's stimulation, they are already panicking about losing their erection or not getting one. Panicky feelings are profoundly antierotic. Trying to stimulate a flaccid penis does not increase pleasure; it is counterproductive, increasing self-consciousness.

Relaxation Is the Foundation

As a man matures, the most important sexual knowledge he must learn is that relaxation is the foundation for sexual response and erection. Men find that idea counterintuitive until they learn that medications like Levitra work by physiologically relaxing the microscopic muscles surrounding the arteries in your penis. That relaxation allows for the dilation of the arteries and facilitates blood flow in your penis. Relaxation and sensual touch are the foundation for sexual response.

Erotic Scenarios

Erotic scenarios involve both partners actively giving and receiving pleasurable touch. Sex is neither a spectator sport nor a proving ground. As a younger man, you may have experienced spontaneous and autonomous erections, but in sexual maturity, conscious or subjective arousal (feeling open, desirous, and turned-on) often precedes and leads to physiological arousal (blood flow to the genitals and penile firmness). A common cause of ED is the lack of direct stimulation to your penis as part of the mutual pleasuring process.

Almost all men prefer to proceed to intercourse on their first erection. Getting into an erotic flow that follows the path of comfort, pleasure, eroticism, arousal, intercourse, and orgasm is highly satisfying. Having intercourse with your first erection becomes a problem, however, if that is the only acceptable scenario and you become self-conscious and panic when there is any variation. We will help you confront your fear of losing your erection and teach you how to get one back easily, let it wane, and then regain it easily. You will learn that as long as you remain physiologically relaxed and stay emotionally open, your erection will be dependable. When you learn how to get, lose, and regain your erection, your self-confidence will return. Then you won't feel you have to prove anything to yourself or your partner, and you can enjoy and accept your sexuality.

■ Jon and Clare

Jon and Clare came to couple sex therapy when Jon was fifty-one and Clare forty-nine. This was a second marriage for both; they had been married nine years. They were committed to making this marriage secure and stable, but Jon's ED was clearly getting worse.

Jon began his sexual life having trouble with premature ejaculation, which is the most common male sexual problem. Jon's rapid ejaculation did not improve over time and was a source of great embarrassment. Yet it did not affect his desire for intercourse. He married at twenty-three, had two children, and was very surprised and hurt when his wife left him seven years later. They were able to coparent successfully, but Jon felt personally and sexually rejected.

He found returning to the dating scene quite stressful, and reacted strongly to a woman's complaint about his premature ejaculation. Jon felt intimidated by the woman's sexual demands. He went to a sex clinic which claimed success with only one consultation. He was put off by the high price and impersonal treatment, but he did receive prescriptions for Viagra to strengthen his erection, an antidepressant at a low dose, and a numbing cream (lidocaine) to delay ejaculation. Did it work? Jon did experience longer intercourse, but he also felt less pleasure and eventually less desire and arousal as well as less connection to the woman.

Jon had his first erectile failure at forty-two. This experience sensitized Jon to fears about his performance. His new worry about erections compounded his old worry over premature ejaculation. Jon felt very sexually vulnerable.

Clare came into Jon's life when his sexual self-confidence was very low. They met at a Parents without Partners group. Clare was the custodial parent of two adolescent children. The year before, her husband had left her for a man. Clare realized he was bisexual but had convinced herself he was dedicated to her and the children. She felt devastated by the loss.

Jon and Clare began as friends, a good way to start a relationship. Jon admired Clare's resilience in reorganizing her life and being the nurturing, stable parent. Clare admired Jon's steadiness and found him to be a nonjudgmental, supportive friend. After four months their mutual attraction was evident, and they became a romantic, sexual couple. From the start, Jon was anxious about sex and apologized for his sexual performance, but Clare felt unconcerned. As long as he didn't have a sexual secret (he didn't), she was sure everything would work out sexually.

Jon and Clare had some special sexual experiences, some good sex, some mediocre sex, and—increasingly—frustrating and dysfunctional sex. Both felt demoralized, but they coped in very different ways. Jon tried to compensate by being the good partner in other ways. He was quite affectionate but avoided sensual or erotic touch. Clare coped by reading simplistic marital and sexual self-help books and encouraging Jon to explore why he was "afraid of sex." Each appreciated that the other's coping techniques were meant to be helpful, but they eventually found themselves frustrated.

Clare purchased an herbal remedy she had read would increase sexual desire, and both she and Jon used it. Clare had a serious allergic reaction and was hospitalized for a night. Learning about the herbal remedy, their internist insisted they not use any medication or other remedy before checking with her. She referred them to Dr. Hwang, a sex therapist with good academic and clinical credentials.

Dr. Hwang explained that sex problems are best approached as a couple and asked Jon and Clare to come in together for the first session. After the first session, Jon and Clare each had an individual session to discuss their psychological, sexual, and relationship background. Dr. Hwang recognized that Jon and Clare had a solid relationship bond of respect and trust and wanted sex to be an energizing part of their marriage. It was clear that ED was a major emotional drain and that Jon's apologizing and blaming himself did not make him an inviting sex partner.

Dr. Hwang pointed out that while optimism and hopefulness are healthy, it is unrealistic to assume that if there is love and communication, sex will take care of itself. Love and communication are necessary but not sufficient to overcome ED. Jon and Clare needed to accept that ED was a chronic, severe problem which would become more draining of their marital bond unless addressed.

Dr. Hwang told Jon and Clare that they would need to develop a new understanding about ED, which would help them work effectively to solve the problem. She outlined a plan which offered hope and motivation to pursue gradual and complex change. Dr. Hwang explained that to facilitate sexual change, they would need to do sexual exercises at home. The first exercise focused on beginning to rebuild comfort with pleasurable touch both inside and outside the bedroom.

To overcome ED, Jon and Clare had to commit to working together and using a variety of resources. Jon got a prescription for Cialis from the internist. He agreed to confront his avoidance pattern by having planned and spontaneous sexual dates two to three times a week. Jon realized that he would have to stop apologizing for himself sexually and instead make sexual requests. Clare decided that she would work to reestablish her "sexual voice." She realized that her sexual responsiveness was good for Jon. Together, they made a *commitment to adopt new expectations about sex and erections and to deal with dissatisfying or dysfunctional experiences without becoming demoralized or giving up (a particularly strong trap for Jon).*

Jon worried that therapy would drag on for months or years. Dr. Hwang assured Jon that couple sex therapy was a focused treatment with a range of ten to twenty-five sessions. As they experienced improvement, they could taper off the sessions with the goal of becoming their own therapists.

Clare made a crucially important point to Jon. His perfectionism was a hindrance to regaining sexual confidence, and she strongly agreed with Dr. Hwang's suggestion that they should aim for good-enough sex (sex that flows to intercourse about 85 percent of the time). Clare was afraid that if Jon needed it to be 100 percent, they would remain in the same cycle, with good experiences being subverted by failures and with Jon being apologetic and avoidant. Although they'd had similar conversations over nine years, this time it made sense to Jon. Clare could be supportive, but it was he who had to stop demanding perfect performance and apologizing when he "failed." For the first time in his adult life, Jon felt he had the freedom to really enjoy erections and non-intercourse sexuality. The comprehensive biopsychosocial approach, combined with a new view of male and couple sexuality, made the difference.

WHAT IF YOU DON'T HAVE A PARTNER?

Although we emphasize sex as a couple issue, we realize there are many men with ED who are single, divorced, or widowed. There are also a number of men whose partners, whether spouses or girlfriends, do not want to see a physician or therapist and view ED as your problem to deal with on your own.

Even if you do not currently have a partner, you do have a virtual partner in the sense that you recall past partner experiences or imagine a partner in the future. You can still benefit from reading and learning about the new model of male sexuality, doing assessments and exercises on your own, and thinking about how you would approach ED issues with a partner. In choosing an appropriate partner, you will want to be sure that the woman is someone you are comfortable with, attracted to, and, most important, who you trust will be a sexual friend in helping you resolve ED.

OUR APPROACH TO OVERCOMING ED

Men ask why ED treatment has to be complex. Isn't there a quick fix? We wouldn't be opposed to easy answers and simple interventions if they worked, but they usually aren't adequate. We want you to do what is right for you. A wise choice is a plan that meets both emotional and practical needs and is successful in both the short and long term. For most men, the wise plan for change addresses physiological, psychological, relational, and psychosexual skill factors. Some men are lucky that just one or two interventions—a medication, a supportive spouse who helps you regain erectile confidence, or a change in sexual expectations—is all that is needed. We encourage you and your partner to read this book, increase your awareness, engage in self-assessments, and complete those steps and exercises that will help to overcome your ED. Make wise choices and use all your resources.

Our comprehensive approach to male sexuality encourages you to treat yourself and your penis in a human way, not as a sex machine. The idea of good-enough sex is difficult for many men to accept, but it is key in maintaining gains and preventing relapse. This guideline is typically easier for the woman to understand and accept because it reflects the reality of her sexual experience. You may worry that aiming for good-enough sex will "feminize" your sexuality or encourage second-class sex, but the opposite is the truth. A variable, flexible approach humanizes male sexuality, is positive and realistic, and gives you the opportunity to enjoy great sex and prevent relapse. Having an erotic, nonintercourse scenario and a sensual, close scenario as backup when sex doesn't flow to intercourse is crucial. Challenge the thought that this is settling for second-class sex. In making these changes in attitudes and couple sexual style, you adopt the principle that the essence of great sex is desire, pleasure, and satisfaction. If you continue to demand that your body perform with 100 percent predictable erections and intercourse, it will result in relapse.

We believe that accurate knowledge is power. You deserve a sexual life that is a positive force enriching all the other aspects of your life. We will provide you with the most up-to-date and helpful information about physiological, psychological, relational, and sexual technique factors to understand ED and to develop your own approach to overcoming ED. This book is not meant to be do-it-yourself sex therapy. If you find that you need the help of a therapist or physician, the appendix to this book,

"Choosing an Individual, Couple, or Sex Therapist," provides guidelines and resources for finding competent professional help.

Here is some basic information to structure your approach to overcoming ED. These concepts and skills will be discussed in detail in the chapters ahead.

- You want sex to again play a positive, integral role in your life and relationship.

- You will learn to understand your ED, assess its cause or causes, plan an approach to overcome your ED, and develop a relapse prevention plan to maintain your gains.

- The keys for satisfying sexuality are for you to adopt realistic sexual expectations; value intimacy; learn relaxed, nondemand pleasuring; integrate eroticism; and develop a variable, flexible couple sexual style.

- We cannot emphasize enough the importance of positive, realistic expectations of yourself and your relationship. It is unrealistic and ultimately self-defeating to try to return to the easy, 100 percent predictable, autonomous erections of your teens and early twenties.

- Maintaining your sexual gains and preventing relapse are just as important as overcoming ED. This is where the comprehensive approach is especially valuable. We see too many men who overcome ED (with or without medication) only to relapse into negative attitudes, behaviors, and feelings about ED and sexuality.

- You are part of a sexual couple, not a perfectly functioning sex machine. Even for men with no history of ED, 5 to 15 percent of their sexual experiences are dissatisfying or dysfunctional. When an erectile problem occurs, you can laugh—or at least shrug off the experience—and make a date to try again in the next one to three days.

- Take pride in having an accepting and resilient attitude toward sex as a couple. You can keep your sexual relationship vital. Continue to make sexual requests and be open to exploring sensual and erotic scenarios.

- The importance of maintaining a sexual relationship that energizes you and gives you special feelings of desirability and satisfaction cannot be overemphasized. Sexuality should not be a deal maker or a deal breaker in a relationship. Sexuality can play a 15 to 20 percent role in maintaining a vital and satisfying relationship. Couples who share intimacy, nondemand pleasuring, erotic scenarios, and planned as well as spontaneous sexual encounters will have a satisfying sexual relationship. That is the major antidote in preventing an ED relapse.

As you begin this work of understanding and changing your ED, be willing to use all your resources to regain comfort and confidence with erections and to enjoy a satisfying couple sexuality.

3

Developing Realistic Expectations about Sex and Your Body

Why should you consider ED as a couple problem? Is this just a trendy concept to hide the truth that you are the man and it is your job to get an erection, have vigorous intercourse, and make sure you last long enough for your partner to have an orgasm during intercourse? Traditional men hold strongly to the myth that a real man can have sex with any woman, any time, any place and that a real man does not need anything from a woman. The new medical variation of this myth is that taking a pill will return you to total sexual performance and self-confidence, again needing nothing from your partner. Old myths about male sexuality give way to new myths. What both types of myths have in common is they burden the man and his penis with a sense of isolation and performance pressure. These myths subvert couple intimacy and negate realistic expectations.

The focus of this chapter is to help you understand and accept your sexual body, how erections "work," and the normal changes in male and female sexual response and sexual function at different stages of life. We will also discuss the impact of physiological conditions such as diabetes, multiple sclerosis, and cancer, as well as sex after age sixty. We encourage you to share information, transitions, concerns, and coping strategies with your partner. Having accurate information is an essential part of challenging sexual myths.

It is easier and healthier to deal with physical and psychological changes together rather than in isolation. This is particularly true of ED, which affects you, your partner, and your relationship. To pretend otherwise is to violate a major tenet of mental health: Do not fool yourself. *ED is truly your common foe.* The likelihood of overcoming ED increases significantly if you work as a team.

The second focus is to develop positive, realistic expectations about erections and sex. It is not enough to label perfectionistic performance standards as unrealistic and self-defeating. The best way to change something is to replace it with new, healthy information and expectations.

THE HUMAN SEXUAL RESPONSE CYCLE

Masters and Johnson (1966, 1970) revolutionized the human sexuality field by describing the physiological sexual response cycle, dividing it into *excitement, plateau, orgasm,* and *resolution.* Kaplan (1974) broadened the model to include a crucial initial stage, *sexual desire.* The complete sexual response cycle consists of five phases: *desire, excitement* (arousal), *plateau, orgasm,* and *satisfaction* (resolution). These physiological patterns are true for both men and women, although the psychological pattern does differ.

Desire

The desire phase involves sexual anticipation, fantasy, and yearning, as well as a sense of deserving sex that is good for you and your relationship, including both physical and emotional openness to sexuality.

Excitement

During the excitement phase, in addition to feeling a subjective sense of pleasure and being turned on, you experience erection and may emit a few droplets of "pre-cum" from the tip of your penis. Women experience increased blood flow to the genitals, vaginal lubrication, breast swelling, and vaginal changes to increase receptivity to intercourse.

Plateau

The plateau phase is when your body's arousal maintains a level of pleasure. If you are physically relaxed, you will maintain pleasurable arousal without quickly moving to orgasm. During the plateau phase, your body "settles in" (becomes saturated with pleasure). Unless there is continual penile stimulation, it is normal for your erection to go down, to "take a break." Not understanding that this is normal, men unnecessarily panic, thinking they have "lost" their erection and it will never come back. This panic is a huge distraction that disrupts the plateau phase and erotic flow. This makes arousal and erection difficult to regain. But with calm relaxation and trust in your body, all that is required is direct, gentle touch to the penis, and your erection will easily come back from its "break."

Orgasm

Sexual pleasure peaks during the orgasm phase and is accompanied by rhythmic contractions of the pelvic muscles and the release of sexual tension. A sensation of ejaculatory inevitability precedes the contractions that result in ejaculation.

Satisfaction

During the satisfaction phase, your body gradually returns to the nonaroused state. Both the man and woman experience a pleasant afterglow, feeling relaxed and sexually satisfied. The afterplay period can be a time of special emotional bonding.

UNDERSTANDING HOW YOUR PENIS WORKS: BASIC PHYSIOLOGY

What is happening when you have an erection is an incredible and complicated process. We want you to appreciate your body and how it functions, and ensure your expectations are reasonable, as well as see the rationale for some of the strategies and techniques we describe (for example, physiological relaxation to promote easy erections).

There are several physical systems that need to function well for an erection.

The Vascular System

A problem with the penile vascular system (blood vessels) is the most common physiological cause of ED. When you are relaxed and open to mental and physical stimulation, blood flow increases to your genitals and specifically your penis. A number of physical, psychological, relational, and situational factors can interfere with this natural increase in blood flow. Common physical causes of ED include vascular disease, high blood pressure, side effects of medication, high blood sugar (poorly controlled diabetes), and vascular injuries. Common psychological factors are anticipatory or performance anxiety, distraction, antierotic thoughts, being a passive spectator, and depression. Relational factors that subvert erectile function include emotional alienation, miscommunication, unresolved conflict, lack of attraction or desire, competition or intimidation, anger, frustration, shyness, or inhibition. Sexual and situational factors which cause dysfunction include lack of privacy to enjoy genital stimulation, trying to have intercourse when minimally aroused, fatigue, not feeling subjectively turned on, and worrying about your partner's anxiety or sexual pain.

The Hydraulics of Erection

Erection occurs when nerve impulses from the brain (*psychogenic* erection) and from genital stimulation (*reflexogenic* erection) combine to cause blood to flow faster into than out of the penis. Your penis is a sophisticated hydraulic system. There are three spongelike cylindrical bodies that run the length of your penis and are fed blood from small branches of the penile artery. These three tubes of spongy tissue swell with blood to cause an erection. Two of these tubes, the *corpora cavernosa*, lie side by side along the shaft of the penis; the third, the *corpus spongiosum*, lies underneath. Together, these three cylinders make up the shaft of your penis.

An erection happens when the microscopic muscles that surround the arteries in the penis relax, causing dilation of the arteries. Blood rushes into the spongy tissues of these cylinders, creating a hydraulic elevation of your penis. Simultaneously, muscles near the base of your penis contract, preventing blood from leaving your penis. For the erection to subside, those microscopic muscles surrounding the arteries stop relaxing and constrict, and the blood in the three cylinders is carried away by the veins that surround them. Most men are surprised to learn that an erection occurs by *physiological relaxation*. This knowledge can help you understand why it is important to learn body relaxation for good erections.

The Chemistry of Erection

The chemistry that manages all this activity is complex. Erection occurs when nitric oxide acts on the smooth muscles surrounding the penile arteries, activating an enzyme which then relaxes the smooth muscles, allowing blood to fill the spongy tissues. An enzyme called *phosphodiesterase type 5* (PDE-5) tries to block this muscle relaxation. The way a medication like Viagra works is to inhibit PDE-5 so that it does not block relaxation. This enhances or prolongs the effect of vascular relaxation and consequently causes erection. A pill doesn't act immediately because it takes some time for the chemical steps to occur and it takes direct penile stimulation to build arousal. On a chemical level, too, it is relaxation (not performance pressure) that facilitates erections.

The Neurological System

A problem with the neurological system is the second most frequent physiological cause of ED. Your nervous system can respond to both mental and physical stimulation to cause your penis to become firm enough to penetrate your partner's vagina. Common neurological problems include disorders like multiple sclerosis, long-term effects of diabetes and other untreated or poorly controlled illnesses, medication side effects, alcohol and drug abuse, and physical injury to the penis. Psychological, relational, sexual, and situational factors can also inhibit neurological function.

The nerves involved in this process connect the lower spine to the penis via the *pelvic nerve*, branching into the *cavernous nerve*, which manages the three spongy cylinders of the penis. The importance of these nerves is evident when damage occurs to this nerve supply during prostate or rectal surgeries, causing postsurgery ED.

From your body's perspective, an erection is a neurological reflex involving the spinal cord and brain. The spinal reflex causes relaxation of the penile smooth muscle, which in turn causes dilation of the penile arteries, resulting in an erection. Numerous higher central nervous system areas in the brain (for example, the *hypothalamus* and *amygdala*) are involved in erections.

The Hormonal System

The hormonal system influences desire and erections through such hormones as *testosterone, luteinizing hormone,* and *prolactin.* Very low levels of testosterone will disrupt sexual desire and functioning. Common causes are a systemic hormonal problem, fatigue and stress, alcohol and drug abuse, or in one case a pituitary tumor.

Understanding better how your sexual body works can help you overcome ED through accurate information and realistic expectations.

MORE ABOUT SEXUAL PHYSIOLOGY

It's useful to understand that the physiological foundation for both men and women is the same. In utero, for the first four to eight weeks, we all were sexually *undifferentiated*—that is, physically neither male nor female. Technically, if no male hormones were introduced, we would all end up female. But with the release of *androgens* triggered by the genetic structure, a male emerges. It's interesting to realize that male and female embryos have similar anatomical and neurological structures. Originally, we all looked female anatomically, having an opening that became the vagina in females or was "sewn shut" in the male. Later, when you are examining your penis and testicles, look for the "seam" down the middle of your testicles. Consider too that your penis is actually a much-enlarged clitoris.

Your Penis's History

Erection is a natural physiological response. Even before you were born, you had spontaneous reflexogenic erections as a fetus. When expectant parents have a sonogram, not only the sex of the fetus but sometimes even an erection can be seen. A newborn boy has his first erection within a few minutes of delivery. And to this day, every night while you sleep, whether or not you're sexually active, you typically have a ten- to twenty-minute natural, physiological erection approximately every sixty to ninety minutes, or three to five erections a night. These erections occur during stage-one REM *(rapid eye movement)* sleep. Physiologically, nighttime erections are your body's way of oxygenating the tissues of your penis to maintain healthy function, and they occur throughout life for men in good health. Truly, you are a sexual person from the day you're born to the day you die.

Getting to Know Your Body and Your Penis

From the moment babies are born, they are fascinated by their bodies. Within your first year, you experience pleasurable sensations by rubbing and stroking your genitals; sexual awareness is born. In childhood, boys and girls examine and compare genitals, playing "house" or "doctor." Looking, touching, and exploring are a part of normal development and promote healthy attitudes toward your body and sexuality.

EXERCISE: Exploring Your Sexual Body

Increase your sexual awareness by engaging in a body exploration, especially of your genital area. Find a time when you have at least thirty minutes of privacy—perhaps the next time you take a shower or bath. A full-length mirror would be helpful, along with a hand mirror. Relax and put aside any thought that this is strange or unnatural. You are taking a good look at your body, and who has more right to do that than you?

Start with your *testicles* ("balls"). Hold them in your hand, using a hand mirror to examine them from all sides. Be aware of their weight and shape. Don't be afraid of hurting them; your testicles are amazingly resilient. The testicles are the principal male sex glands, and they house the *seminiferous tubules* where sperm are manufactured. In addition, the testicles manufacture testosterone, which affects male physical characteristics (like hair and beard growth) and sexual desire. So efficient are the testicles that if one is removed (for example, to treat testicular cancer), the remaining testicle is adequate for sexual and reproductive function.

Sperm are created by the millions in your testicles. Sperm travel through the *epididymis* tubes inside the testicles, where they become mature. Sperm leave the testicles by way of the *vas deferens*, two soft, thin tubes that lead into the *seminal vesicles*, storage chambers for the sperm, and then into the *prostate*. It is in the prostate that the sperm are mixed with seminal fluid called *semen*, the whitish, alkaline liquid that spurts from your penis during ejaculation. Sperm are extremely tiny, contributing only 3 percent to the total volume of the ejaculate. Thus when the vas deferens is surgically closed off in a *vasectomy*, only sperm are left out of the mix. A man who has had a vasectomy continues to ejaculate semen as before, with no decrease in force, amount, or pleasure.

The testicles are housed in a bag of loose, wrinkled skin called the *scrotum*. One testicle usually hangs lower than the other. The scrotum can contract or relax, at times allowing your testicles to dangle freely against your thighs and at other times drawing up into a neat, tight package. Notice the "seam" made when the tissue was joined in utero to form your scrotal sack. This is the same tissue that forms part of the lips of the *vulva* in a woman. The scrotal muscles come into play during sexual excitement. When aroused, a man's testicles rise in his scrotum and increase in size. If arousal does not culminate in ejaculation, the swelling remains, causing an uncomfortable sensation of prolonged fullness, popularly known as "blue balls." This is temporary and causes no damage.

Emerging just above the scrotum is the base of your penis. The *shaft* of your penis is the "barrel" and extends from the base to its top or "head," called the *glans*. This is the most sensuous, erotic part of your penis, containing an extremely high concentration of nerve endings. A particularly sensitive area of the head is the ridge at its base, called the *corona*. Areas of greater sensitivity vary according to your experiences and feelings. Some men, for example, find the penile shaft particularly responsive to stimulation.

Most men have thought about and handled their penis, exploring the sensations. It is the focus of intense emotions; few men regard their penis dispassionately. You may be proud of it, ashamed of it, anxious about it, even afraid of it. But a man experiencing ED inevitably feels frustration or other negative emotions about his penis. Clear your mind of preconceived notions and look at your penis as if you have not seen it before.

The erotic stimulus for your erection may come from your brain, via sexual thoughts and fantasies, or from direct physical touch. The first kind of erection (called psychogenic, spontaneous, or automatic) is common in younger men. As you become older—about thirty-five or forty—an erection will ordinarily require direct stimulation to your penis. This is not an indication you are developing ED, but is a natural change with aging which can enhance sensation and pleasure.

Now that you have taken time to explore your penis, have a good talk with your partner. How do you remember feeling about your penis before ED? Proud? Anxious? Shy? Embarrassed? Confident? "Cocky"? Did you appreciate your penis or take it for granted? Then reflect on how you have been feeling about your penis since ED. Confused? Disappointed? Numb? Angry? Frustrated? How can you and your penis become friends (again)?

The Myth of Penis Size

Ideas about male sexual anatomy and physiology have been dominated by superstition and misinformation. Men stubbornly perpetuate penis myths because they are afraid to challenge sexual folklore of what it means to be a "real man." The most destructive myth, which continues to exert a powerful negative influence in spite of scientifically established fact, concerns penis size. Penis size differences (or, more precisely, *perceived* differences) are the basis for an enormous amount of male anxiety. It is true that there are differences in size of the flaccid penis, but that has little to do with penis size or sexual functioning in the erect state. There is no relationship between penis size and ED. The average penis is between two and a half and four inches in the flaccid state and between five and a half and six and a half inches when erect. The diameter is about one inch flaccid and one and a half inches when erect. It is more meaningful to say a normal penis is of proper size to function during intercourse. This definition includes almost all men.

Interestingly, three of four men (75 percent) believe their penis is smaller than average (Jamison and Gebhard 1988). Besides being statistically impossible, this illustrates how the performance-machine model dominates male sexuality, leaving men to feel anxious and insecure. Psychological and relational health is promoted by adopting a positive body image, which includes accepting your penis. Remember, there is no scientific relationship between penis size and sexual desire or response for either the man or the woman. A relaxed, erotic, flexible sexual style is more important than size for pleasurable sex.

A related myth is that a large penis results in the woman being orgasmic during intercourse. This is based on the mistaken belief that the vagina is the woman's major sex organ. In truth, the woman's most sensitive genital organ is her *clitoris,* a small, cylindrical organ located at the top of the vaginal opening where it joins with the *labia* ("lips") of the vulva. The clitoris has a multitude of nerve endings, like the glans of your penis only concentrated in a much smaller area. It is the focal point of her sexual pleasure. Most women prefer gentle, peripheral clitoral stimulation, whether with your hand, tongue, or penis.

During intercourse the clitoris is stimulated by pulling and rubbing action caused by pelvic thrusting—stimulation which is independent of penis size. The vagina, which is in contact with the penis, has fewer nerve endings, most of which are in the outer third. Moreover, the vagina is an active rather than passive organ, which means the vagina swells and expands with her arousal to engage your penis, and can adjust to the penis whatever its size. It usually takes ten to twenty minutes of pleasuring for the vagina to fully expand. If a couple is rushing to intercourse, the man may mistakenly think that his penis is too small, as intercourse does not feel snug. The remedy for this is enjoying pleasurable touch and genital stimulation before intercourse to allow her body to reach the plateau stage of arousal, when her vagina has expanded. Sexual incompatibility based on the couple's genitals is, with extremely rare exceptions, a myth.

YOUR PARTNER'S SEXUALITY

Both men and women follow a similar physiological arousal sequence, although the psychological and relationship factors are somewhat different.

A New Model of Women's Sexual Response

Basson (2001) has described that in committed, long-term relationships, a woman's sexual desire becomes more integrated into her psychological system. Basson notes that in the beginning phase of a new relationship, romantic love and passionate sex lead to easy sexual response for women, but in a long-term relationship (after one or more years), increased distractions and fatigue lead to a different kind of sexual response.

In this model of female desire and sexual response, women have a lower biological urge for the release of sexual tension than men. Orgasm is not necessary for satisfaction and does not need to occur at each sexual encounter. Basson proposes that women's sexual desire is often a responsive rather than spontaneous event, greatly influenced by subjective psychological excitement. While a man's sexual desire may be energized by physical drive, typically a woman's sexual desire develops from her receptivity to gentle, relaxed sensual touching. This touching leads to sexual desire and continues to emotional closeness, affection, sensuality, and eroticism. Sexual desire can develop *after* initial sensual contact. Healthy female sexual response in an established relationship begins in sexual neutrality, but sensing an opportunity to be sexual, his desire, or one or more potential benefits that are important to her and their relationship (for example, emotional closeness, bonding, love, affection, healing, acceptance, or commitment), she elects to seek sensual contact and stimulation. With beginning physical arousal, she may become aware *at that time* of desire to continue the experience for *sexual* reasons and experience more arousal, which may or may not include wanting orgasm. This brings her a sense of physical well-being with added emotional benefits. This model acknowledges that sexual desire for men may be more biologically driven while for women it may be more psychological and relational.

Understanding Your Partner's Reaction to ED

Basson's view of a woman's sexual response offers an understanding of why many women eventually become frustrated, hurt, angry, or avoidant at experiencing ED lovemaking. If ED distracts her partner or stalls the sexual interaction, not only is the sensual value of sex frustrated, but more importantly the flow of intimacy is disrupted. This is exacerbated when you stop lovemaking because of your frustration, apologize, and "go away" emotionally or physically. Sex, which is substantially about emotional closeness, becomes abandonment.

This understanding of your partner's sexuality can help you both become more accepting and respectful of each other's sexual experience. This gives you context and motivation for learning to stop negative reactions to your ED and to cooperate as a team. Men commonly feel physical and sexual frustration at not ejaculating due to ED. Too often, men mistakenly think that ED is a *sexual* frustration for the woman rather than an *emotional intimacy* frustration. It is less about your sexual performance and more about shared closeness and emotional intimacy. Most women strongly value personal attention, touch, and your presence. Don't let ED block this.

Learning to Be a Sexual Lover

Lovers are made, not born. Your ability to enjoy sex and make sex enjoyable for your partner is dependent on your comfort, awareness, psychosexual skills, sensitivity, imagination, and ability to communicate—all of which are a matter of learning and experience. You can increase awareness of your potential as a lover and learn how truly satisfying sex can be if you transform performance-oriented sex to pleasure-oriented sex. Sexuality integrates your personal feelings about yourself as a man, including your attitudes, emotions, behavior, body image, values, physical well-being, and—most important—how you feel about your relationship. At its essence, sexuality is an interpersonal process.

■ Juan and Julia

Thirty-seven-year-old Juan had been divorced for eight years, and he now felt ready to commit to a serious relationship. However, he was very worried and embarrassed about his ED. Juan first experienced ED at twenty-eight. It began abruptly and was the first cue that there was a problem with his marriage. Unfortunately, Juan interpreted his ED as a physical problem. His answer was to intensify his exercise regimen and add an exercise to try to strengthen his erections. This could have been a good strategy except for two factors. First, he missed the major cause of his ED, which was his wife's growing emotional alienation from Juan and the marriage. Second, rather than focusing on exercises that would emphasize body relaxation, identifying and relaxing pelvic muscles, and practicing the wax and wane of his erection, Juan tried to strengthen his penis by keeping it erect as long as he could. That exercise made no physiological or psychological sense. Over the next year, Juan bought four or five products from Web sites that featured glowing personal testimonials and "guaranteed" him longer, stronger erections, but these did not help.

Juan believed the cultural myth that divorce happens when men leave marriages after twenty years for a younger woman. (In fact, divorce is highest in the first two years, and it is usually the woman who leaves because she is disappointed in the man and the marriage.) Partly because he believed that myth, Juan was devastated by the ending of his marriage. He blamed the ED and obsessed about his ex-wife having sex with other men.

Most of Juan's sexual experiences over the next eight years involved masturbation, where he felt in control and had good erections. His occasional sexual encounters were of the "hooking-up" variety. Usually sex occurred late at night after too much alcohol and was often—although not always—unsuccessful.

Juan and Julia met when both volunteered for a community improvement project. Juan was very attracted to Julia, but he was afraid to talk to her about sex. He did not get an erection the first time they tried to be sexual. Juan made sure Julia was orgasmic through oral stimulation but said nothing to her about his sexual feelings. Julia was both open-minded and psychologically inclined, and she was worried about Juan's silence and avoidance. Two days later, Juan took Viagra and they had a successful, although quick, intercourse. Julia hoped that after a successful experience, Juan would be more willing to discuss sexuality issues. Juan was tentative but did disclose how his sense of worth was shaken by the divorce. He told Julia that he very much wanted this relationship to be successful and felt that taking Viagra would ensure a good erection. Julia felt touched and assured Juan that she too wanted a satisfying intimate and sexual relationship. Juan was much relieved and wanted to leave it at that, but Julia realized one loving talk would not be enough.

Julia wanted to develop a close, trusting relationship with Juan and work with him to understand and confront the ED. She wanted a sexual relationship where both felt comfortable and confident with arousal and erection. Julia had taken a human sexual behavior class in college. (Women are much more willing than men to enroll in sexuality classes and read sexuality books.) As a twenty-one-year-old senior, she had experienced men with premature ejaculation but not ED. However, she did learn from the lectures and readings that by age forty, 90 percent of men had at least one experience when they did not get or could not maintain an erection sufficient for intercourse. She wanted to share this knowledge with Juan and be supportive. She didn't like the idea of Juan depending totally on Viagra and panicking each time they were not able to have intercourse.

Julia bought a male sexuality book for Juan (we list a number of these books in the Resources section) and encouraged him to read what was relevant for him. She let him know that she was open to his sexual ideas and requests. Juan was daunted by the idea of objectively assessing the physical, psychological, relational, and psychosexual skill factors contributing to his erectile problems and then developing a change plan. He was won over by Julia's observation that if they did this now, they wouldn't have to be afraid of ED in the future. When Juan got his Viagra prescription renewed, he asked the doctor whether there might be some kind of disease or medical problem contributing to his ED. The physician assured Juan that he was in excellent health. He didn't ask Juan any questions about his relationship, and Juan didn't bring it up, but the doctor told Juan not to worry since the Viagra was working.

Julia was more of an extrovert and more of an optimist than Juan. His tendency was to keep his own counsel and be an anxious worrier. Julia encouraged Juan to share more with her. As they processed emotional and sexual ideas together, Juan found these topics less frightening.

Juan's approach to a serious relationship was highly ambivalent. He very much wanted Julia in his life but felt closeness was not "manly." Julia was not a dependent person, but she did want a serious relationship that had the potential to lead to marriage and a family. While Julia was not desperate to marry, she wanted to give this relationship a good-faith effort. She wanted them to approach ED as a mutual challenge. She did not consider ED to be a reason to break off the relationship, nor did she consider overcoming ED a prerequisite to continuing the relationship. Their most important discussions involved erotic scenarios and techniques. Juan viewed Viagra as a way to short-circuit the need for erotic stimulation. He wanted just enough genital stimulation to allow for an erection firm enough for intercourse, and then he wanted to go for it. Julia felt that Juan was walling her off sexually, cheating them of the pleasures of sexuality, and undercutting their erotic potential. Julia enjoyed intercourse and could be orgasmic with manual, oral, and intercourse stimulation. She valued intimacy, pleasuring, playfulness, and eroticism and didn't want Viagra to substitute for these. Juan worried he would feel sexually intimidated by Julia, but she reassured him these were requests to increase involvement and pleasure, not performance demands. Juan said he was willing to go to a couple therapist, but Julia suggested that they first try on their own.

Over weeks and months, Juan and Julia explored intimate, pleasure-oriented, and erotic sexuality. Gradually, Juan weaned himself from using Viagra, but kept it as a backup in case there were two to three unsuccessful experiences in a row. Juan did not want to regenerate anticipatory or performance anxiety. Julia was clear that when stimulation did not flow to intercourse, she was very happy to share nonintercourse erotic sex or warm, cuddly time. Juan realized that these were special sexual experiences and did not overreact when intercourse did not occur. Together, Juan and Julia had made their sexual relationship a source of pleasure and closeness.

ADAPTING YOUR SEXUALITY TO CHANGING REALITIES

Your sexuality is an essential aspect of your personal development as a man. It is integral to who you are. As you adjust to the changing events and situations in your life, your sexuality also needs to adapt.

Adapting to the Normal Changes with Aging

Contrary to popular mythology, aging does not cause ED and does not stop you from being sexual (Moore et al. 2003). What is true is that normal aging and illness can alter your sexual response. So you and your partner need to be willing to accept and adjust to normal sexual changes. For most couples, this means putting more emphasis on sexual cooperation, increased time spent with pleasuring, and adding erotic scenarios and techniques. In other words, you compensate for decreases in physiological efficacy by creating psychological, relational, and sexual efficacy. With aging, sexuality can become more intimate and interactive, and ultimately more human and satisfying. The more you (and your partner) understand and accept normal bodily changes, the healthier and more satisfying your couple sexual relationship.

For example, with normal aging, your vascular and neurological systems respond more slowly and with less intensity. Therefore, sexual arousal requires a greater degree of relaxation and focus on pleasure, more direct penile and erotic stimulation, piggybacking your arousal on your partner's arousal, being open to her guiding intromission, and being open to nonintercourse scenarios.

The following list summarizes some of the changes thought to be normal with aging.

- Morning erections decrease in frequency.

- There is a mild decrease or no change in sexual desire (sex drive).

- Mental arousal mellows in intensity, perhaps due to subtle neurological changes.

- To obtain an erection (after age thirty-five or forty), direct penile stimulation is usually required; desire is not sufficient to initiate erections.

- Delayed erection is normal, presumably because of mild, decreased penile sensitivity due to changes in neural thresholds. It may take two to three times longer than in youth (that is, five to thirty seconds) to *begin* erectile response. With fatigue, obtaining an erection may take even longer.

- Erections may be less firm, and for some men over sixty, full rigidity may occur only seconds before ejaculation. This is called *ejaculatory surge*.

- Some men may be able to maintain an erection for a longer period of time prior to ejaculation, a benefit to men with a history of premature ejaculation.

- Ejaculatory urgency ("the need to ejaculate") may be reduced. Many men do not ejaculate each time.

- The sense of impending orgasm may be muted. Ejaculation may be single-staged as ejaculatory inevitability is not as well defined.

- Ejaculation may last for only two to four seconds (instead of three to ten seconds in younger men), with one or two ejaculatory expulsive contractions of the urethra (instead of the three or four major contractions in youth), and have reduced intensity (strength of expulsive force). Some older men may have no prostatic contractions with ejaculation (semen may "ooze out"). Orgasm without ejaculation is normal.

- After ejaculation/orgasm, detumescence (going down) of your penis and testicular descent are more rapid due to the decreased amount of blood trapped in the spongy tissues of your penis.

- The refractory period (time before you are able to regain an erection and ejaculate again) increases in length. When you're in your twenties, the refractory period is minutes; when you're over fifty-five, it may be twelve to twenty-four hours or longer.

These are subtle changes, often unnoticed, and usually easy to adapt to if you have reasonable expectations of your body. Some changes are even beneficial, such as the slowed ejaculation for the man with premature ejaculation.

Adapting to Illness

As we age, the prevalence of illness increases, especially high blood pressure, heart problems, or diabetes. An example of adapting to illness is adjusting to the effect of cancer treatment on sexuality and erections. Of course, each type of cancer, treatment protocol, and stage of treatment will affect sexual response differently. The following guidelines apply to most illnesses. First, be a knowledgeable and active patient. Second, talk to your physician (ideally with your partner present) about possible sexual effects of the disease and treatment, and how to cope with these. You want to maintain sexual intimacy, even if that means temporarily stopping intercourse (for example, right after surgery). You will need to communicate with your partner in order to maintain a flexible sexual relationship. Often, the physician will offer a medication like Viagra, Levitra, or Cialis. You need to know what to expect physiologically and consider how you can integrate the medication into your couple sexual style. Remember that within the biopsychosocial model, a limitation in any factor (in this case, biological) can be compensated for by emphasizing another factor (psychological, relational, or psychosexual skills).

Adapting to the Side Effects of Medications

A major cause of ED is unintended side effects of prescription and over-the-counter medications. This is a particular concern of aging men (and women), who are often taking multiple medications. It is important that you let your physician know about sexual side effects and discuss strategies to address them.

DEVELOPING POSITIVE, REALISTIC SEXUAL EXPECTATIONS

To regain solid confidence with your erections, you need to pilot yourself with realistic expectations. You can't expect more of your body (and especially your penis) than it is biologically built to do. This exercise will help you develop healthy, realistic expectations about sexuality, erections, and intercourse.

EXERCISE: Evaluating Your Sexual Expectations

What do you expect from your sexual life? How does this compare to what actually happens with other men and couples? What are positive, realistic expectations? At the beginning of each section, ask yourself what your expectations are. If you are part of a couple, ask your partner to do this exercise too. Write down your responses; this makes them more concrete.

1. **Frequency**

   How often do you expect to have sex? What influences this: the quality of your relationship; your body's urges; the balance of work, childcare, and leisure time? Do you and your partner agree on frequency? What does it mean if you are having less, or more, sex than you expect?

   Most couples do not spontaneously agree on how often to have sex, which presents an opportunity for you to cooperate for mutual satisfaction. The average sexual frequency for married couples is between four times a week and once every two weeks. Contrary to popular belief, married couples are more sexually active and satisfied than couples who are dating or living together. For couples in their twenties, average intercourse frequency is two to three times a week, and for couples in their fifties, it is once a week (Michael et al. 1994). Couples who are sexual less than twice a month may find it hard to develop and maintain erectile confidence. You'll have the most success if you establish a regular sexual rhythm.

2. **Arousal and Erections**

   In what situations do you find it easy to get an erection? When is it more difficult? What does it mean when you have difficulty getting an erection? What does it mean when your erection wanes before or during intercourse? If arousal does not flow to intercourse, what kind of backup plan is acceptable to you? When you don't have an erection sufficient for intercourse, are you and your partner comfortable with erotic, nonintercourse sex to orgasm for one or both of you?

3. **Intercourse**

   What are realistic expectations about intercourse? How have you determined this? Do you expect that each time you have any genital touch, it will result in intercourse? What does it mean to have good-enough erections and intercourse? How do you know when you are "cured"?

One key is to maintain the focus on sharing pleasure before and during intercourse. In other words, if you're both satisfied with the pleasure you're giving and receiving, you have a solid foundation for your sexual relationship. Another key is seeing intercourse as a mutual, interactive experience. If arousal flows to intercourse 85 percent of the time, will you feel good about couple sexuality? Will your partner?

4. **Satisfaction**
    What do you require to feel emotionally and sexually satisfied? Must you experience intercourse and orgasm? Should each encounter be equally satisfying? Why is a mediocre or dysfunctional sexual experience distressing for you? Do you think that "servicing sex" (making sure your partner has an orgasm) is okay? Complete the sentence *I am wonderfully sexually satisfied when* . . . .

    Even among well-functioning, satisfied married couples, half or fewer of their experiences are equally satisfying to both partners. In fact, if you have one or two experiences a month of movie-quality sex, you can count yourselves very lucky. Perhaps 20 to 25 percent of sexual experiences are very good for one partner (usually the man) and good for the other. Another 15 to 20 percent are okay but not remarkable. The most important thing to understand is that 5 to 15 percent of sexual experiences are mediocre, dissatisfying, or dysfunctional (Frank, Anderson, and Rubinstein 1978). Remember, this is true of well-functioning, satisfied couples.

EXERCISE: Negotiating Positive, Reasonable Sexual Expectations

Now that you've each examined your own expectations, you'll want to discuss these and try to come to mutually acceptable understandings about sexual expectations that fit your preferences and relationship. This can be a challenging and difficult process. Take your time. Try to be open-minded and communicate in a respectful, caring manner. It is normal and even healthy to have differences; you are not clones of each other. If you find your expectations are very different or you cannot communicate and reach an understanding, you may want to seek help from a therapist (see the appendix to this book, "Choosing an Individual, Couple, or Sex Therapist," for suggestions).

- How often do you expect to have sex? What generates your sexual desire? What is a comfortable frequency that fits your need for connection?

- How long do you expect pleasuring (foreplay) to last? Intercourse? What about the time is most important and meaningful to you? Can you agree on a range of time which is comfortable and satisfying for you both?

- How comfortable are you accepting that it is normal for your erection (or her vaginal lubrication) to come and go during a pleasure-oriented sexual interaction?

- What are your preferences for intercourse? Do you enjoy slow, sensual intercourse? Do you prefer fast, intense intercourse? What are your preferences regarding multiple stimulation during intercourse?

- In what percentage of sexual experiences do you expect your partner to be orgasmic? Do you (and she) have preferences for her being orgasmic during manual, oral, rubbing, or intercourse stimulation? Can you accept variability?

- What determines your satisfaction with your sexual experience? Is it possible to feel satisfied without intercourse or orgasm?

- What percent of the time do you expect sex to be great, what percent satisfactory, what percent all right? Can you accept a poor quality sexual experience? What do you think is reasonable?

- How do you each want to handle times when sex is dissatisfying or dysfunctional?

WHAT YOU CAN EXPECT FROM OUR MODEL

In the same way it is important to have reasonable expectations of yourself and your body, it's important to understand what you can expect from our approach. You will *not* become a teenage sexual performance machine with 100 percent guaranteed erections. You *will* regain confidence with erections and enjoy a pleasurable and satisfying couple sexual style. You *will* enhance your relationship by learning to share and value a variable, flexible couple sexuality that integrates intimacy, pleasuring, eroticism, arousal, intercourse, and afterplay.

Learning a new approach to erections and couple sexuality is like learning any other skill. It is a gradual process requiring persistence, patience, and practice to change attitudes, learn new psychosexual skills, and cooperate as intimate friends. An interested, involved, and aroused partner is the best aphrodisiac. You and your partner can utilize all of your resources (medical, psychological, relational, and sexual) to learn and maintain confidence with erections and sexuality.

The essence of erectile confidence involves developing realistic expectations, learning to physically relax your body, being open to pleasure-oriented touching, being receptive and responsive to giving and receiving genital stimulation, getting into an erotic flow, experiencing intercourse as a natural continuation of the pleasure-eroticism process, being open to your partner's taking an active role (which can include guiding intromission and engaging in multiple stimulation during intercourse), and enjoying the afterplay process. Comfortably switching to an erotic, nonintercourse scenario or a sensual, close scenario is a crucial coping strategy when sex does not flow into intercourse. Remember, the essence of great sex is desire, pleasure, and satisfaction.

4

The Causes and Effects of Erectile Dysfunction

After years of functional erections and enjoyable sex with Sarah, Tom was stunned when he experienced ED. He literally panicked inside, feeling unsettled, baffled, embarrassed, anxious, and frustrated. To "fail" at sex after years of good functioning, he assumed the cause had to be serious. He reasoned that only a significant cause could yield such a profound physical failure. He worried that something was seriously wrong, but what could it be? He felt aggravated that his penis had betrayed him when he needed it to perform. But what was the cause? Was the cause profound? Or was it something simple that would cure itself? Was he physically ill? Did it mean he was losing his sexual desire for Sarah? Was there a problem with their relationship? Why was Sarah so supportive at first but now so quiet? He felt disoriented and at a loss about what he could do. He wondered whether one of the new erection medications (maybe Levitra or Cialis) could be the solution.

THE MULTIPLE CAUSES, DIMENSIONS, AND EFFECTS OF ED

There are many causes for ED. In this chapter we will help you understand the complexity of what can at first look like a fairly clear-cut and straightforward problem. You will need to look deeper than simply observing what is going wrong with your penis. Real-life problems are rarely simple, easy to solve, or magically fixed, in spite of quick-fix promises.

While the experience of ED is pretty much the same for all men—difficulty getting or keeping an erection sufficient for intercourse—there are actually ten different types of ED. Causes of ED fall within four general groups: physical, psychological, relational causes, and those stemming from psychosexual skills deficits.

In addition to understanding the multiple causes of ED, it is important to appreciate that ED is multidimensional. There is an interaction between the physical, psychological, relational, and psychosexual skills dimensions. For example, ED that results from a vascular problem (physical) may influence your self-esteem (psychological), affect communication with your partner (relational), and even influence your feelings about work (psychological). This intermingling and intertwining of the facets of our personalities and lives is normal. There is also a subtle intermingling of your and your partner's thoughts, feelings, and behaviors, which adds to the complexity. This is why ED can feel so confusing, so difficult to sort out.

It's not just the causes and dimensions of ED that are complicated. The effects or consequences are complicated too. ED can have a devastating impact on your self-esteem, your sex life, and your relationship. These effects, in turn, make ED worse. It's a vicious cycle.

In this chapter we will help you understand all of the possible causes of ED and explain the multiple dimensions that can make ED seem so confusing, as well as illuminate the negative effects that ED may have on you and your relationship. The psychological and relational features are particularly complex and intertwining, so we'll offer you a model to help you understand how these dimensions fit together and how to develop a change plan. Then, in chapter 5, we'll help you determine the causes of your ED so that you'll be prepared to develop a comprehensive and effective approach to remedy your ED.

To illustrate these interacting dimensions, consider the following example. (We identify each relevant dimension in parentheses.)

■ Phil and Sandi

Phil was twenty-six years old, married for four years to Sandi, with a two-year-old son and an established, satisfying career as a teacher. Phil and Sandi's sexual relationship was one of the strengths in their marriage, and they took considerable pride in maintaining a satisfying sex life amidst the responsibilities of family and work. So when one night Phil could not get an erection, he and Sandi were baffled (psychological). He felt irritated with his penis—it seemed to betray him (biological and psychological)—and uncharacteristically powerless, not knowing what to do (psychological and psychosexual). He was at a total loss (psychological) to know how to handle the intrusion into their love life (relationship). His mind searched for reasons (psychological): maybe there was something wrong with his body (biological, medical)?

Did this mean his relationship with Sandi was in trouble (relationship)? Was his difficult childhood catching up to him (psychological)? Could his ED result from his now seeing Sandi more as a mother than as a lover (psychological, relationship)?

Were his recent challenges at work upsetting him more than he realized (psychological)? Was his ED somehow related to two earlier lovemaking sessions when he ejaculated too fast (psychosexual skills)? Was he simply fatigued from work stresses and parenting (psychological and physical)?

With the help of assessment and intervention strategies, Phil and Sandi were able to understand and sort out the problem and resolve ED. You can do it, too.

THE "BIG FOUR" TYPES AND CAUSES OF ED

ED may be caused by extensive and complicated factors or by subtle and seemingly insignificant ones. While there may be one cause for your ED, commonly there are several occurring simultaneously to produce and maintain ED, with reverberating effects on your personal well-being as well as your relationship.

To help you understand the possible causes of your ED, we'll consider the "big four" groups. The *physical* group of causes includes physiological system problems, medical illnesses, physical injuries, personal lifestyle risks, and drug side effects. The *psychological* group is composed of psychological system characteristics and individual psychological distresses. The *relational* group involves difficulties in relationship identity, cooperation, and emotional intimacy. In the *psychosexual skills* group, ED results from a lack of cognitive, emotional, or behavioral skills or from using these skills ineffectively. Be aware that what may cause or maintain your ED may also be an effect of it. For example, distressing relationship conflict may cause ED, but it may also be a consequence of ED caused by another factor.

In classifying the types and causes of ED, it is helpful to distinguish two dimensions of ED: the onset and the context. The onset of ED distinguishes between *lifelong* ("primary") and *acquired* ("secondary"). The vast majority of ED experiences are acquired; that is, ED develops after a period of satisfactory erections. The context of ED distinguishes between *global* (occurring in all situations, including masturbation, and with all sexual partners) and *situational* (occurring in some situations but not others: for example, with a partner but not during masturbation, with one partner but not another, or during intercourse but not oral sex). These two features—onset and context—will help you sort out what type or types of ED you have.

The Physical Types and Causes of ED

Let's begin by considering the physical types and causes of ED.

Physical System ED

Physical system ED involves physical, structural, or neurological barriers to adequate sexual function and erections. This cause of ED is rare, and this type of ED is inevitably lifelong. *Congenital* or biological structural features can limit the body's sexual function. Among the several conditions that are considered to be predominantly biologically determined is *gender identity disorder*, a very rare condition that may sometimes manifest with an ED problem. This is an internal conflict between one's psychological and biological gender (for example, male-to-female transsexualism). More common is *paraphilia* (for example, transvestism), which is considered at least in part a biologically limited arousal pattern. Here, the individual experiences difficulty with desire and arousal because his physical system is programmed to feel aroused by various impersonal contents (for example, women's clothing).

Brain studies in animals and studies of twins (Bailey and Pillard 1995) as well as genetic studies in humans (Pillard and Bailey 1995) suggest that *sexual orientation* (attraction to the opposite sex, same sex, or both sexes) has roots in the neurological system. Scientifically, homosexual or bisexual orientation is considered a normal variant (Cabaj and Stein 1996). However, when a man with same-sex orientation denies his innate sexual attraction to men (for example, fearing societal stigma if discovered) and tries to perform heterosexually, ED may result.

While some consider physical age a cause of ED, we do not. You will hear about studies that conclude that age is the strongest predictor of ED. The misleading factor here is that these studies do not take into consideration physical illnesses and side effects of medications. The more accurate conclusion is that as men become older, they have more significant, chronic illnesses and are more likely to be taking medications. It is not aging that causes ED, but rather illness and medication side effects.

Medical Illness ED

Illness may cause acquired ED that typically occurs in all sexual situations. A number of acute diseases are known to cause ED. Some are common illnesses, such as diabetes and high blood pressure, while others are very rare. Illnesses that affect the vascular, neurological, hormonal, and muscular systems have the potential to hinder or even block erections because of their role in sexual response (Segraves and Balon 2003). Because sexual response relies on these multiple physical systems, virtually any illness may include ED as an effect.

Physical Injury ED

Temporary or permanent damage to your body that directly or indirectly affects the vascular, neurological, hormonal, or muscular systems can cause ED. For example, ED results from spinal cord injuries, trauma to the perineum ("biker's ED," where intense, prolonged bike riding may cause harm to the perineal vascular or neurological system), or damage caused by penile *priapism* (erections lasting more than four hours). Common causes of ED are surgeries (such as cardiac surgery, radical prostatectomy, spinal cord surgery, or cystecomy) and pelvic area radiation and chemotherapy for cancer treatment.

Lifestyle Issues ED

There are several lifestyle factors that are known to cause or contribute to ED. The most common lifestyle cause of ED is alcohol consumption (see the next section). Long-term smoking or passive exposure to smoke may cause ED by harming the penile vascular system. Obesity or a sedentary lifestyle with poor physical conditioning may limit the physiologic responses of arousal (for example, respiration and cardiovascular efficiency).

Another common lifestyle cause of ED is fatigue. Excessive work or exercise (for example, marathon training) can stress your body. Fatigue is a common cause of ED among middle-aged and older men, although younger men can also experience ED when excessively fatigued. Couples typically engage in sex late at night, when fatigue is most common, after a day of work, anxieties, and family requirements. ED resulting from such lifestyle issues is acquired, occurs intermittently, and can occur in all sexual situations.

Drug Side-Effect ED

ED may occur as a side effect of certain drugs. The most common cause of ED in men younger than forty is excessive alcohol consumption. By forty years of age, most men have had at least one episode of ED, often the result of alcohol misuse. In spite of the subjective feelings of lowered inhibitions, alcohol is technically a central nervous system depressant, which means that it restricts the functioning of the neurological system.

There are a number of prescription and over-the-counter medications that may cause ED as a side effect (Schatzberg and Nemeroff 2004). Medications to treat high blood pressure, antihistamines (for colds or allergies), cancer chemotherapies, and some psychotropic medications (for depression or anxiety) are among the more common agents, although any medication may be suspected until you can rule it out. Drug side-effect ED is acquired and occurs in all sexual situations.

The Psychological Types and Causes of ED

Your brain is your major sex organ, and detrimental thoughts, feelings, and experiences can cause ED.

Psychological System ED

Psychological system ED is caused by chronic psychological problems such as obsessive-compulsive disorder, chronic depression (dysthymia), generalized anxiety disorder, bipolar mood disorder (manic-depression), schizophrenia, a personality disorder (for example, avoidant personality disorder, dependent personality disorder, or borderline personality disorder), post-traumatic stress disorder (the aftereffects of witnessing tragedy or being victimized), or developmental disorders such as attention deficit/hyperactivity disorder; by the ongoing psychological effects of alcoholism or drug abuse; or by chronic, unresolved personal issues (especially those involving sexual guilt or shame).

While significant psychological problems can cause ED, scientific studies reveal that the vast majority of men with ED do not have a major psychological problem, nor do they share a common personality profile (Weeks and Gambescia 2000). This type of ED might not manifest in men in their twenties or thirties but usually does occur throughout the man's life and in all sexual situations.

Psychological Distress ED

Psychological distress ED is caused by temporary psychological difficulties such as an adjustment disorder (for example, anxiety or depression in reaction to specific situations or events such as loss of job). Nearly 50 percent of the population will experience a psychological distress situation sometime in life (Amen 1998). Another factor, such as physical illness ED, can cause psychological distress because anxiety and stress distract from the sexual situation. Often it is difficult to determine whether the psychological features are the cause or result of ED. Psychological distress ED is acquired and usually occurs intermittently. It is more common and is easier to address and change than psychological system ED.

Men tend to underestimate the effect that psychological stress can have on their sexual functioning, assuming that when there is such a profound problem as ED, the cause must be profound as well. In fact, it does not take much psychological distress to disrupt sexual functioning. ED is more likely when the man has situational anxiety, reactive depression, loss of confidence, doubt, disappointment, irritation, remorse, embarrassment or negative feelings about his body, unrealistic expectations of sexual performance, or experiences internal conflicts such as between the roles of lover and father (Fagan 2002). In addition, losses (death of a parent, friend, loss of income), midlife adaptations, changing social status, parenting stresses, monotony, reaction to your partner's distress, and even success can disrupt your psychological function.

Psychological distress not only may *cause* ED but is almost invariably an *effect* of ED. Most men with ED feel at least mild inadequacy, discouragement, self-doubt, or anxiety.

Psychosexual Skills Deficit ED

Psychosexual skills deficit ED results from absent or ineffective cognitive, emotional, or behavioral skills related to lovemaking. The man does not have accurate and sufficient knowledge about his body, his partner's body, and sexual physiology (how sexual response works); has a number of distorted cognitions (thoughts or beliefs); has unreasonable expectations about sexual performance; and lacks essential sensual skills for arousal. Some men also lack interpersonal skills such as talking warmly of sex, making sex comfortable, and cooperating with a partner to achieve sexual satisfaction. This type of ED is lifelong but commonly does not occur with masturbation because the man feels more comfortable and less self-conscious when he masturbates.

The Cognitive-Behavioral-Emotional (CBE) Model

To help you understand the multiple dimensions of the psychosexual skills aspects of ED, we offer you a framework: the *cognitive-behavioral-emotional* (CBE) model. This will help you make sense of the otherwise confusing experience of ED and organize your approach to overcoming your ED.

The CBE model recognizes that each individual is composed of *cognitions,* or thoughts; *behaviors,* or actions; and *emotions,* or feelings. These experiences comprise the "core discussion" you have with yourself as well as your action plan to deal with the situation.

Cognitions or Thoughts

Cognitions involve ideas, beliefs, assumptions, observations, perceptions, interpretations, and expectations. These are unique to each person. Cognitions are beneficial or detrimental depending on their effect on your feelings and actions. Appreciate that your thoughts powerfully drive your feelings. Your thoughts about your sexuality—beliefs, standards, perceptions, expectations, and assumptions—are vital to your sexual response and satisfaction. This is why we are so careful to remind you that your sexual expectations must be solidly grounded on a reasonable view of your body, sexual response, and your sexual relationship. You want to reinforce reasonable and positive thoughts; don't set yourself up for frustration and failure.

Behaviors or Actions

We choose to act (or not act) based upon our thoughts and feelings. Action is always a decision. The freedom to choose your behavior may be constrained by thoughts and feelings, but responsible and mature living mandates accountability for your behavior. Behaviors may be constructive or destructive depending on their effect on the individuals and the relationship.

Emotions or Feelings

Emotions are chemical-electrical "energy" events or experiences in your body. You label this energy according to how you experience these physical sensations: fear, sadness, loneliness, dread, satisfaction, resentment, worry, contentment, frustration, pleasure, irritability, excitement, anxiety, surprise, confusion, shame, guilt, comfort, embarrassment. Feelings are "motivators" that prompt, penalize, or reward action. Feelings are not themselves good or bad, right or wrong. Feelings influence the thoughts we have and the actions we take. Emotions are described as positive or negative depending on how you subjectively experience them and how they influence your behavior. You will need to understand and manage your feelings so they do not disrupt your efforts to change.

Thoughts, feelings, and behaviors interact in a complicated web of influences—thoughts influencing feelings, feelings influencing behaviors, and behaviors prompting thoughts and feelings. For example, you may expect (cognition) that you will "fail" (cognition) to get an erection, feel frustration (emotion), and anticipate (cognition) that your poor performance (behavior) will cause your partner's disappointment (emotion). Making love with this predisposition, you will have difficulty focusing (cognition) on your pleasurable sensations; become preoccupied (cognition) with anticipating erectile failure; have difficulty relaxing (behavior) your body; lack awareness (cognition) of techniques (behavior) to facilitate erections; become preoccupied (cognition) by your partner's body and reactions (behaviors); experience restricted, uneasy, or anxious sensuality (emotion); or entertain distorted thoughts (cognitions) such as *I must have an erection or she will leave me.*

While these features work against you in this example, recognize that you can make them work for you by replacing negative cognitions, behaviors, and emotions with realistic, beneficial ones. In the CBE model, each component is valued and is integral to promoting change. Understanding the cognitions, behaviors, and emotions that contribute to your ED will help you overcome the problem.

Relationship Distress ED

Complicated relationship dynamics (for example, failure to communicate, unresolved emotional conflicts, mistrust in response to infidelity) may cause ED, maintain ED caused by a different factor, or result from ED. The CBE model focuses on three fundamental dimensions of intimate relationship satisfaction: relationship identity, cooperation, and emotional intimacy.

Relationship Identity

Relationship identity refers to the composite *cognitive* life of your relationship—the beliefs, attributions, and expectations that each of you brings to your relationship; the relevance of your personal history; and what your relationship means to each of you. For example, how do you balance needs for individual autonomy and relationship cohesion? In healthy relationships, each individual benefits from the relationship, and the relationship benefits from the input of each individual.

Relationship Cooperation

Relationship cooperation refers to your composite *behavioral* interactions—how you communicate, work together in a balanced way, and solve problems in an effective and mutually agreeable manner. Your thoughts and feelings are hidden from each other unless you communicate them through a behavior, typically by discussing them. This is why communication is such an important part of couple sexual growth.

Relationship Emotional Intimacy

Relationship emotional intimacy refers to your relationship's "environment" or quality of *emotional* bond. Intimacy includes the emotional, friendship, and sexual aspects of your relationship—feelings of affection, commitment, and closeness.

Deficits in these relationship features undermine the mutual emotional acceptance that is so important to healthy sexual functioning. Even when ED is caused by something other than relationship distress, it can cause considerable damage to your relationship. Relationship distress ED is acquired and limited to sex with your partner.

■ Darin and Leticia

When Darin first struggled to obtain an erection, Leticia reacted uncharacteristically with anger, blaming him for ruining their sex life. She relied on their lovemaking as a way to escape the burdens of being a mother to their two grade-school children and the pressures of her career as a medical clinic office manager. To not be able to enjoy sex regularly and satisfactorily felt like having the rug pulled out from under her.

Darin was stunned by her hostile reaction. They were not the kind of couple who fought or expressed strong negative feelings—until his ED. He pulled away, feeling responsible for Leticia's distress and mortified by his failure. He could not accept that his penis had failed him, nor could he believe that Leticia could be so angry with him.

Darin's withdrawal continued outside the bedroom. Leticia noticed his subdued manner, and she felt embarrassed by her automatic, irritable behavior in the bedroom. They each gingerly went about their "business" of parenting and work. Each felt punished by the other, and resentments began to develop. After four days of subdued avoidance, Leticia finally broke the ice awkwardly, asking Darin in a detached tone of voice, "What's wrong?"

Darin automatically interpreted her question as What's wrong with you? and reacted defensively. "You're what's wrong!"

The blame and counterblame went on for only a moment, but the emotional hurt was deep and lasting.

To make things worse, their younger child developed strep throat that required Leticia to stay home until the antibiotics took effect. "More stress," she complained when Darin arrived home that evening, and another argument ensued. Each became more frustrated with the other, with one negative exchange cueing another.

Darin and Leticia had avoided sex since the night Darin had trouble getting an erection, and after ten days, Darin masturbated "to see if it still worked." He was alarmed when he once again could not get an erection. He tried and tried until he was incredibly frustrated and turned off. Thinking that he must have some physical problem, he set up an appointment with his family doctor.

His doctor immediately suspected the prescription antihistamine Darin was taking for allergies, although the medication was only infrequently associated with ED, according to the pharmaceutical company's clinical trials. His doctor suggested stopping the medication and going several weeks without an antihistamine to see if his ED would self-correct. If it did, his doctor would prescribe a different medication that would not cause ED.

Although still hypersensitive, Darin shared with Leticia the discussion he'd had with his doctor. Each was skeptical and not eager to try sex again. Darin's performance anxiety so paralyzed him that they didn't have sex until six days after he stopped the antihistamine, when Leticia gently initiated one night. He was reluctant at first, fearing failure and another painful exchange. However, Leticia gently stroked his chest and stomach for ten minutes. He gradually lowered his apprehensiveness, appreciating Leticia's gentle approach. He opened to her touch and began to caress her arm and shoulder, and with patience and mutual pleasuring, he began to gain an erection. Although each felt tentative, they made love in a way that was somewhat distant but ended in a feeling of great relief.

The next day, they cautiously talked about what had occurred the night before. Maybe it was simply the medication that was the culprit. Maybe the medication—combined with the ordinary stresses of work and family and the fatigue of that late night—had caused his ED and set off the painful relationship conflict. Maybe. They decided to have sex again that night to "test it out." Again, it took some patience and cooperation, but they enjoyed their lovemaking, this time with less distance and more pleasure.

Over time, they regained mutual comfort, pleasure, and satisfaction in their sexual relationship. Sex was once again a major source of sustenance. Darin was prescribed an alternative antihistamine that did not cause ED. They discussed their realization that Darin's ED was probably caused by the combination of the medication and fatigue, and that their frustration, blame, and counterblame was a regrettable mistake which exacerbated the problem. Each learned from the experience. Leticia learned to not personalize Darin's *sexual response difficulty; Darin learned to stay engaged with Leticia when he was sexually anxious. While a very painful experience, ED helped them to grow as an intimate team.*

ED with Another Sexual Dysfunction (Mixed ED)

ED coexists with another sexual dysfunction (such as low sexual desire, premature ejaculation, or ejaculatory inhibition) about one-third of the time (Loudon 1998) and can reflect a combination of physical and psychological causes. For example, a vascular cause for ED may combine with psychological and relationship distress to create a loss of sexual desire. Occasionally, men try so hard to prevent premature ejaculation that they unintentionally cause ED, which can lead to inhibited sexual desire. Treating the premature ejaculation can, in turn, help resolve the ED. In addition, your reaction to your partner's sexual dysfunction (such as low sexual desire, inhibited arousal, sexual pain, or nonorgasmic response) can cause or exacerbate your ED.

YOU CAN UNDERSTAND YOUR ED

In the next chapter, you will engage in an assessment process to determine the cause or causes of your ED. If you determine that your ED has a single cause, that is good. However, it is more likely that there will be multiple causes, dimensions, and effects. The intermingling of these features—physical (medical, hormonal, vascular, neurological), psychological (cognitive, behavioral, emotional), relational (identity, cooperation, intimacy), and psychosexual skills deficits—can complicate your effort to understand your ED and plan how to overcome it. Nevertheless, you can address all these important factors.

Your efforts will be good enough; you do not need to be perfect to overcome your ED. By being comprehensive and inclusive, you can overcome feelings of helplessness and hopelessness, develop the tools to regain comfort and confidence with erections, and cooperate with your partner to enrich your sexual relationship.

5

Assessing Your Erectile Dysfunction

In this chapter, we will help you answer several important questions about your ED. What are the criteria that differentiate ED from healthy sexual functioning? What type of ED do you have? What are the causes? How severe is your ED? How can you develop a comprehensive, individualized approach to resolve your ED?

When you determine the causes and severity of your ED, you take the most important step on the road to resolving your problem. You know what you are dealing with and can set a course of action—individually and as a couple—to overcome your ED.

DO YOU HAVE ED?

ED is the consistent, dissatisfying experience of being unable to obtain or maintain an erection sufficient for sexual intercourse. You have ED if your erectile capacity is inconsistent or insufficient and this is distressing to either you or your partner. Consider the following six questions:

1. Can you get an erection most of the time (in at least four out of five sexual experiences) when you receive direct penile stimulation?

2. Can you keep an erection for more than five minutes (when you want to) in at least four out of five sexual experiences?

3. Are you able to comfortably enjoy the pleasure in your penis rather than monitor your penis to make sure you have an erection and will succeed at intercourse?

4. Are you able to relax well enough to enjoy pleasure and eroticism during lovemaking?

5. Are you able to feel close and connected during intercourse?

6. After you and your partner make love, are you both usually pleased and satisfied?

If you are not able to answer yes to these questions, you are experiencing the common features of ED. On the other hand, if you answered yes to all of these questions, you do not have ED. If you answered yes to all but still feel that you have ED, you need to reevaluate your sexual expectations so they are reasonable in terms of physiological function and relationship intimacy.

HOW SEVERE IS YOUR ED?

Evaluating the severity of your ED will help you decide how detailed, deliberate, and determined you will need to be in developing and completing your change plan.

EXERCISE: Erectile Dysfunction Severity Index (EDSI)

Circle the number that indicates what you typically experience for the questions below.

1. How long has ED been a problem for you?

10	9	8	7	6	5	4	3	2	1	0

Lifelong   Intermittent   Recent
                   ("off and on")   (less than
                                          one year)

2. In what percent of all sex acts are you *unable* to obtain or maintain an erection?

10	9	8	7	6	5	4	3	2	1	0
100%	90%	80%	70%	60%	50%	40%	30%	20%	10%	0%

3. When does ED usually occur?

10	9	8	7	6	5	4	3	2	1	0

Unable to get erect   Get erect but it soon goes away   Lose at penetration   Lose shortly after some intercourse

4. If you can have intercourse, how long is it before you typically lose your erection?

10	9	8	7	6	5	4	3	2	1	0
As you enter	15 sec	30 sec	1 min	2 min	3 min	4 min	5 min	6 min	7 min	More than 7 min

5. Rate the intensity of physical stimulation at the time you lose your erection.

10	9	8	7	6	5	4	3	2	1	0

Very intense, vigorous, or fast   Moderate stimulation   Very mild, little, or slow

6. How difficult is it for you to initially get an erection?

10	9	8	7	6	5	4	3	2	1	0

Extremely difficult   Moderately difficult   Extremely easy

7. How upset is your sexual partner when you lose your erection?

10	9	8	7	6	5	4	3	2	1	0

Extremely distressed   Moderately upset   Very calm

8. How upset are you when you lose your erection?

10	9	8	7	6	5	4	3	2	1	0

Extremely distressed   Moderately upset   Very calm

9. How much has your ED negatively affected your life in general?

10	9	8	7	6	5	4	3	2	1	0

Major impact (for example, ruined relationship)   Some impact   No significant effect

10.   What percent of the time when you have ED do you also have low
       sexual desire, premature (rapid) ejaculation, or delayed (inhibited)
       ejaculation?

10	9	8	7	6	5	4	3	2	1	0
100%	90%	80%	70%	60%	50%	40%	30%	20%	10%	0%

Scoring the EDSI

To determine your severity index, add your responses to items 1
through 10 and enter your total score in the appropriate category below.

_____ *0–19 Very mild*

_____ *20–39 Mild*

_____ *40–59 Moderate*

_____ *60–79 High*

_____ *80–100 Extreme*

The lower your severity score, the more likely you are to successfully resolve your ED. The more severe your ED, the harder it will be to
remedy and the more disciplined you and your partner will need to be. If
your case is of moderate severity, you have a good chance of addressing
ED successfully through the techniques in this book, but you will need to
invest a good amount of personal and relationship energy. If your score
indicates high or extreme severity, it is very likely you would benefit
from the coaching and support of a trained marital and sex therapist. See
the appendix to this book, "Choosing an Individual, Couple, or Sex
Therapist" for guidelines.

DEVELOPING YOUR INDIVIDUALIZED PLAN

In order to overcome ED, you will need to be determined and patient.
You will need to use all your resources. You may need to develop a more
comfortable, cooperative relationship. You may need to find a wise and

affirming physician for a medical evaluation. You may need to consult with a skilled and knowledgeable marital and sex therapist. Decide as a team your individualized approach to resolve your ED. Congratulate yourself for having the courage to face this difficult problem.

Using Your Personal Diagnostic Team

Begin the process by assembling your personal diagnostic team.

Your Partner

You want your partner to be your strongest support. Ask for her help. She will be reassured that you want to operate as a team in improving your sexual relationship. Going through the diagnostic process together will create a comprehensive picture and be very useful later as you cooperate to address your ED.

Your Physician

The physician is the professional most men prefer to talk to about sexual concerns. You may find it awkward to initiate the discussion, but remember that doctors usually take their cues from the patient. If you do not bring up your concerns, your doctor probably won't either. So go ahead and initiate the discussion. It helps to mentally rehearse what you will say:

> Dr. Miner, I am having trouble with erections. I am embarrassed to ask about ED, but I need your help. Can you help me with my sexual concern?

Your doctor may not have special training in sexual medicine, but he or she will certainly want to help you understand ED and decide on medical interventions if warranted.

This exercise will help you decide whether you should see your physician for a physical examination. Your doctor can rule out medical problems or simply reassure you. Take the lead and ask your doctor to look for physical causes of your ED. Even if there is not a physical cause, your physician is an excellent resource for identifying sexual medicine or sex therapy professionals who can join your personal diagnostic team.

EXERCISE: Do You Need a Medical Evaluation?

1. If your age is

    younger than thirty years, have you had a full physical exam within the past five years?   Yes   No

    thirty to forty-four years, have you had a full physical exam within the last four years?   Yes   No

    forty-five to fifty-nine years, have you had a full physical exam within the last two years?   Yes   No

    older than sixty years, have you had a full physical exam in the last six to twelve months?   Yes   No

2. If you responded yes to the physical exam question, did your exam include

    complete medical history and review of systems?
    Yes   No

    physical examination of your body?   Yes   No

    physical examination of your genitals?   Yes   No

    laboratory test of complete blood count (CBC)?
    Yes   No

    Did the physician know about your sexual concerns?
    Yes   No

3. Is your general health very good or excellent?   Yes   No

4. Is the medical history of your immediate family (parents, siblings) free of significant medical or genetic problems such as diabetes, vascular disease, heart disease, cystic fibrosis, thyroid or other endocrine problems, obesity, or neurological problems?   Yes   No

5. Is your health good enough that you do not take medication (except a vitamin supplement) regularly?   Yes   No

If you have answered no to any item above, a medical evaluation may be wise. Be sure to tell your physician you are concerned about ED and want careful evaluation and testing, not just a pill.

DETERMINING THE CAUSES OF YOUR ED

To understand and remedy ED, it is crucial that you determine its cause or causes and its effects. Do not conclude that the first cause of ED is the only one. Continue through each of the ten steps in order to determine all of the possible causes, effects, or manifestations. You want to be inclusive, because if you miss a cause or effect, you will overlook a potentially important factor in your change plan. Don't allow yourself to fail by an oversight.

EXERCISE: Determining the Causes of Your ED

As you follow these ten steps, note your answers on the summary sheet that follows.

Step 1: Do you have physical system ED?

Yes   No   Has ED occurred all your life?

Yes   No   Has ED occurred in all sexual situations (with different partners, during masturbation)?

Yes   No   Do you have a biological system problem that can cause ED, such as a congenital genetic, neurologic, hormonal, urologic, or gender dysphoria problem?

If you answered yes to all of these, you may have physical system ED. It is not easy to conclusively diagnose physical system ED until you have a detailed medical evaluation. This is a very rare cause of ED.

Step 2: Do you have medical illness ED?

Yes   No   Has your ED been acquired (developed after a period when you had adequate erections)?

Yes   No   Does your ED occur in all situations?

Yes   No   Did the previous exercise indicate that you need a physical examination?

Yes   No   Do you have a family history of vascular, endocrine, renal, or neurological irregularities?

Yes   No   Do you have or think that you could have one of these illnesses:

diabetes mellitus	sleep apnea	Peyronie's disease
multiple sclerosis	hypopituitarism	hypogonadism
hypothyroidism	systemic lupus	sexually trans- mitted disease (STD)
polyneuropathy	chronic renal	
lipid abnormalities	failure	
cardiac disease	vascular disease	epilepsy

If you answered yes to the first two items and at least one additional item, it is possible that you may have medical illness ED. You will need a complete medical evaluation to determine whether a physical illness might be causing or contributing to your ED. This is a common cause of ED.

Step 3: Do you have physical injury ED?

Yes   No   Has your ED been acquired?

Yes   No   Does your ED occur in all situations?

Yes   No   Has there been a physical injury, surgery, or trauma which preceded or coincided with ED? Such injuries could include spinal cord injury; head injury; trauma to the pelvic area (including trauma caused by intense or excessive bicycling); trauma to the penis; priapism; surgery to the abdomen, chest, pelvis, or colon; prostatectomy; or chemotherapy.

If you answered yes to these questions, you may have physical injury ED. If you suspect an injury may have caused your ED, consult with your family physician. This is an infrequent cause of ED.

Step 4: Do you have lifestyle issues ED?

Yes   No   Has your ED been acquired?

Yes   No   Does your ED occur intermittently or frequently?

Yes	No	When you experience ED, have you consumed alcoholic beverages within the previous several hours?
Yes	No	Are you significantly sleep deprived?
Yes	No	Do you now smoke, or have you previously smoked?
Yes	No	Are you now overweight and have you been for more than one year?
Yes	No	Are you aware of being exhausted or fatigued more days than not?

If you answered yes to the first two questions and at least one additional item, you may have lifestyle issues ED. It would be wise for you to address the issue with your physician or other health-care professional. This is a common cause of ED.

Step 5: Do you have drug side-effect ED?

Yes	No	Has your ED been acquired?
Yes	No	Does your ED occur in all situations?
Yes	No	Are you taking a cardiovascular or hypertension medication known to cause ED?
Yes	No	Are you taking a medication known to cause ED, such as an antihistamine, antispasmodic, neuroleptic, antianxiety medication, antidepressant, gastrointestinal drug, prostate cancer medication, antiseizure medication, or diuretic medication?
Yes	No	Are you using a "recreational" drug, such as MDMA ("ecstasy"), cocaine, alcohol, or methadone, known to cause ED?
Yes	No	Did your ED begin at or shortly after the time you began taking a new drug or medication of any type (including over-the-counter)?

If you answered yes to the first two items and an additional item, you may have drug side-effect ED. Remember that while many medications may have a negative effect on your sexual functioning, the dosage and combination with other medications you take is very important. This is the most common physical cause of ED. If you suspect drug side-effect ED, be sure to discuss your concerns with your physician or pharmacist.

Step 6: Do you have psychological system ED?

Yes   No   Has ED occurred all your life or at least since age twenty-five?

Yes   No   Has ED occurred in all or most partner situations?

Yes   No   Have you been diagnosed with—or do you think you have—a serious, lifelong, chronic psychological character pattern or unrelenting problem such as obsessive-compulsive disorder, chronic depression, generalized anxiety disorder, or dependent personality disorder?

Yes   No   Do you have an immediate relative (sibling, parent, grandparent) who has a chronic psychological character pattern or unrelenting psychological problem?

Yes   No   Do you have a sexual arousal pattern with strong interest in sexual objects or situations (such as fetishism or exhibitionism) that may significantly limit your ability to get sexually excited during couple sex?

Yes   No   Do you think you are naturally more aroused by same-sex subject matter or persons (homosexuality) *and* are you trying to function within a heterosexual relationship?

Yes   No   Have you taken a formal psychological test that suggests you have a chronic psychological problem?

If you answered yes to the first two questions and one other, you may have psychological system ED. While psychological system ED is rare, it is important to consider this because if you do not address the underlying cause, your efforts to remedy ED will be unsuccessful. Careful evaluation will help sort out the extent to which the psychological problem must be treated in order to resolve your ED.

Step 7: Do you have psychological distress ED?

Yes   No   Has your ED been acquired?

Yes   No   Does your ED occur in all or most partner situations?

Yes   No   Are you experiencing significant worry or anxiety; sadness, depression, or grieving; frustration or resentment; or profound self-doubt or discouragement in reaction to a major life event such as a death in the family, marital infidelity, unemployment or career change, sudden success, the birth of your child, or moving your residence?

Yes   No   Does your partner have a psychological problem (such as obsessive-compulsive disorder, major depression, generalized anxiety disorder, or a personality disorder) to which your ED may be a reaction?

Yes   No   Have you taken an objective psychological test that verifies you are experiencing current psychological stress?

If you answered yes to the first two items and at least one additional item, you may have psychological distress ED. The critical difference between psychological system ED and psychological distress ED is its source and severity. Psychological distress ED is a reaction to life events and is usually easier to treat. This is a common cause of ED.

Step 8: Do you have psychosexual skills ED?

Yes   No   Has ED occurred all, much of, or on and off throughout your life?

Yes   No   Has ED occurred in most situations, especially with a partner?

Yes   No   Do you focus your sexual attention almost exclusively on your partner—her body, actions, sexual response?

Yes   No   Are you so distracted that you are unable to physically relax during sex or unable to focus on the pleasure of your own sensations?

Yes   No   Do you feel confused about your sexual response and perplexed about how to work with your body to obtain and maintain your erection?

Yes   No   Are you shy about asking your partner for what you want during sex?

Yes   No   Do you initiate and anxiously pursue sex with highly arousing activities such as oral-genital sex or immediate intercourse rather than beginning slowly with relaxed kissing and light massaging?

Yes   No   Do you have detrimental thoughts or beliefs about sexual functioning such as *I must have an erection or she will be disappointed, ED means that I am a complete failure,* or *To be a good lover, I must give her an orgasm during intercourse?*

Yes   No   Do you react to your ED with negative behavior such as apologizing, acting irritable, blaming (yourself or your partner), withdrawing or retreating, or other inflexible or uncooperative behaviors that disrupt your lovemaking and closeness?

If you answered yes to the first two items and several others, you may have psychosexual skills ED. This type of ED is common.

Step 9: Do you have relationship distress ED?

Yes   No   Has your ED been acquired?

Yes   No   Does ED occur only with your partner?

Yes   No   Has your partner recently expressed dissatisfaction with your general relationship?

Yes   No   Are you experiencing difficulties in balancing autonomy and cohesion (relationship identity issues)?

Yes   No   Are you experiencing difficulties in cooperatively resolving relationship conflicts (relationship cooperation issues)?

Yes   No   Are you or your partner acquiescing to avoid conflict and unintentionally holding resentments (relationship cooperation issues)?

Yes   No   Are you experiencing a deficit in emotional empathy (relationship emotional intimacy issues)?

Yes   No   Have you recently taken an objective test that suggests relationship distress?

Yes   No   Have you thought recently that marital or relationship therapy might be helpful?

If you or your partner answered yes to the first two plus at least one other question, you may have relationship distress ED. Relationship distress ED is distinguished by acquired onset and situational occurrence in partner sex. It is a common cause of ED.

Step 10: Do you have ED with another sexual dysfunction (mixed ED)?

Yes   No   In addition to ED, do you experience another sexual problem (low or inhibited sexual desire, premature ejaculation, difficulty ejaculating during intercourse, or ejaculating without an erection) more than 25 percent of the time?

Yes   No   Does your partner experience inhibited sexual desire, nonorgasmic response, *dyspareunia* (pain with intercourse), *vaginismus* (reflexive constriction of the vaginal muscles making penetration painful or impossible), or other significant discomfort (for example, lower back problems) to which your ED may be a reaction?

If you answered yes to one of these items, you may have ED with another sexual dysfunction (mixed ED). It is normal to have sexual difficulties on occasion, but when this occurs regularly, it represents a sexual dysfunction. Successful treatment of the other sexual problem can help resolve your ED.

EXERCISE: ED Self-Evaluation Summary Sheet

As you work through the previous exercise, mark the types of ED you think you may have. Where applicable, list the specific cause you suspect.

☐   Physical system ED
     (what condition? _____)

☐   Medical illness ED
     (what disease? _____)

☐   Physical injury ED
     (what injury? _____)

☐   Lifestyle issues ED
     (what lifestyle condition? _____)

☐   Drug side-effect ED
     (what medication or drug? _____)

☐   Psychological system ED
     (what condition? _____)

☐   Psychological distress ED
     (what distress? _____)

☐   Psychosexual skills ED
     (what skill or skills? _____)

☐   Relationship distress ED
     (what area or areas of distress? _____)

☐   ED with another sexual dysfunction (mixed ED)
     (what other dysfunction? _____)

Your summary sheet offers a comprehensive view of the areas you'll need to address in your action plan to resolve your ED. If you think you may have a physiological type of ED, a medical checkup will help you confirm this. If you think you may have a psychological or relationship type of ED, a psychological consultation may help you confirm this.

SUMMARIZING WHAT YOU KNOW ABOUT YOUR ED

Now that you have completed the summary sheet, review with your part- ner your findings on the causes of your ED as well as your EDSI score from the "How Severe Is Your ED?" exercise earlier in this chapter. What does your EDSI score tell you about how determined you will need to be to resolve your ED?

ORGANIZING YOUR TREATMENT APPROACH

Based on the causes and the severity of your ED, you now can decide on resources and strategies to change it. Approaches to overcome physically caused ED (physical system, medical illness, physical injury, lifestyle issues, or drug side-effect ED) are described in chapter 6. Treatments for psychologically based ED (psychological system, psychological distress, or relationship distress ED)—and strategies for repairing individual and rela- tionship damage from ED caused by other factors—are described in chap- ter 7. Interventions for psychosexual skills ED are described in chapter 8. The approaches we describe in chapters 7 and 8 can also help you adapt to physically based ED, enhance sexual satisfaction, and prevent relapse. Now that you have identified all the elements contributing to your ED, you can confidently engage in addressing these elements—and succeed!

6

Medical, Pharmacologic, and Physiological Treatments

In this chapter, we explore the medical treatments that are available for ED. We discuss several approaches to reverse ED caused by necessary medications like antihypertensive drugs. We offer you balanced information about Cialis, Levitra, and Viagra, and we discuss how to use them in a way that enhances intimacy rather than as a quick fix. In addition, we describe treatments such as the penile vacuum device and surgical implants, as well as experimental surgery for penile vascular disease. We offer recommendations for what *not* to do. We discuss the pros and cons of each option in terms of personal pleasure and relationship satisfaction as well as effectiveness in treating ED.

ADDRESSING THE MEDICAL SIDE OF ED

ED that originates from a biological cause needs treatment that addresses the physiological problem, or you will face disappointment and frustration in your attempt to overcome your ED. Remember, you want to address all the factors involved in your type of ED and use all your resources— including medical treatment, medication, and physiological aids.

The Fix-and-Foster Principle

There is a two-part guiding principle for treating physical ED: fix and foster. After the physical cause is "fixed," the couple will need to heal from the distress ED caused and use relationship and psychosexual skills to recover cooperation and foster sexual intimacy and satisfaction. Your physician is trained to alleviate biological problems when possible but does not have the power to ensure relationship satisfaction. That is your job! "Fixing" the medical cause of your ED does not itself foster sexual and relationship satisfaction. Don't settle for less.

Medical Treatment Can Help Treat Psychological ED

Medical treatments can also be used to help when a psychological cause blocks your sexual progress. When out-of-control performance anxiety causes or maintains ED, you may use an oral medication to do an end run around the anxiety. The medication works together with your psychological effort to lessen your anxiety. Medication acts as an "insurance policy" to help you reestablish your sexual confidence. Gradually, you can taper off the medication as your performance anxiety is alleviated.

Your Relationship Is Your Home Base

As you weigh the medical options available to you, remember to return "home"—to your partner, your intimate relationship—to make your decisions. While any medical decision is an individual choice, remember that because it affects your sexual relationship, it is also inherently a relationship decision. Consider and respect your partner's feelings and preferences. Ask her view, remembering that two heads are better than one. Research on the effectiveness of surgical penile prostheses ("implants") established that while surgical implants are technically effective in achieving erections, the ultimate effectiveness—satisfaction—largely depended on whether the sexual partner accepted the intervention (Sidi, Reddy, and Chen 1988). In too many cases, when the partner was not involved, surgery would create a good erection, but it had no place to go. Remember that sex is not so much about performance (erections) as it is about sharing pleasure and intimacy. Taking a pill may technically produce a fine erection, but does it guarantee sensitivity and cooperation in the bedroom? Keep your perspective. Your relationship is home base.

What's Involved in a Medical Evaluation

Your general physician (whether an internist or family practitioner), who knows you and your medical history best, is the likely first choice to discuss your sexual concerns. Medical evaluation for ED typically consists of three steps.

History. Your physician will ask you about your personal and family medical history and talk with you about your experience of ED. This will include discussing general medical background, basic information about when and how often you experience ED, a brief sexual history, other physical symptoms, your ideas of the cause, and how distressed you are. Your doctor is trying to gain a comprehensive understanding of your situation as well as rule out various medical causes.

Physical Examination. During a thorough evaluation, your doctor will examine your body, focusing on your genital area, and may check your penis and testicles as well as your genital nerve reflexes.

Testing. Blood and urine tests may be done to make sure there is no systemic problem. The blood pressure in your penis may be taken using a small blood pressure cuff. Laboratory testing may include testosterone levels, serum glucose, and lipid profile. These tests are probes for problems in the endocrine, vascular, and neurologic systems.

A trial of an oral medication (for example, Cialis or Viagra) is a reasonable diagnostic approach. This test can help determine if your vascular system is sufficient. If medication does not help, your doctor may refer you for consultation with a urologist. The urologist's evaluation may include injection testing that can help differentiate physical from psychological ED. Injection testing may be combined with penile ultrasound, which offers a nonintrusive look inside your penis to evaluate its vascular system. Normal findings suggest ED may be caused by neurologic, hormonal, or psychological factors. Specialized tests such as cavernosometry, cavernosography, arteriography, or nocturnal penile tumescence studies (using a portable machine at home to monitor your erections during sleep) may be helpful in evaluating ED.

■ Derek and Susan

Derek, a thirty-eight-year-old accountant, and his wife Susan, a thirty-four-year-old social worker, felt profound fatigue trying to keep up their careers, care for three young children (eight, six, and three), and help an elderly neighbor attempting to remain independent. So when Derek began to have trouble getting and keeping his erection, emotional fatigue seemed the likely culprit. At first they tried to ignore the sexual problem, but as ED became more frequent, it was more distressing.

After several weeks, they had a very painful exchange. Derek told Susan she was too passive and said, "You save no energy for me!" Susan shot back, "You only care about your dick! What about me?" Later they realized that arguing was counterproductive, apologized, and vowed to avoid a repeat of the conflict. Unwittingly, they prevented a reoccurrence of the argument by avoiding sex. Derek was perplexed by his ED, while Susan attributed it to the stresses and pressures of their daily lives. She felt stressed to the maximum, and now the negative sexual undercurrent added to her burden. To have ED seemed to fit the overwhelming responsibilities they felt.

Derek's ED varied but persisted. He and Susan attempted sex only infrequently, less than once a month. An ad on TV urged Derek talk to his doctor about ED, and he took this suggestion. He asked his doctor for "a sample of that sex pill on TV," which the doctor provided. At the same time, the doctor wisely conducted a brief screen for medical problems and noted Derek had a family history of hypertension and diabetes. His blood pressure was normal, so a blood sugar test was scheduled to determine if Derek's ED could be an early symptom of diabetes. Derek was relieved when the results were negative. Cialis was effective in improving Derek's erections, and he and Susan gradually regained their sex life.

At a follow-up medical appointment, Derek told his doctor that Cialis worked fine but that sex was still very infrequent because he felt so fatigued most of the time. Prompted by questions from his physician, Derek listed his lifestyle stresses and recalled that Susan had at times commented that he snored badly and seemed to gasp for air during sleep. Suspecting a sleep problem as a source of Derek's fatigue and low sexual desire, the doctor ordered a sleep study. Sleep lab findings confirmed that Derek had moderate to severe sleep apnea, and he was prescribed a machine to aid his breathing during sleep.

After several months Derek was feeling better, and he wanted to try sex without the medication, buoyed by his morning erections. He was pleased— and relieved—to function well. He and Susan gradually found themselves being playful again at sex. Their lives were still very stressful, but sexuality was a positive refuge, not a further source of stress.

Derek's ED was multicausal, stemming from detrimental cognitions (*You save no energy for me!* and *You only care about your dick!*), his general level of emotional and physical stress, and the physical fatigue resulting from lifestyle demands and sleep apnea. Understanding these multiple causes and effects helped Derek and Susan to confront ED effectively. Derek later thanked his doctor, appreciating his thoroughness in helping Derek understand and treat his ED.

TREATMENTS FOR PHYSICAL SYSTEM ED

If your responses to the exercise in chapter 5 suggested you may have physical system ED, you should have a thorough medical evaluation by a knowledgeable physician. While this cause is very rare and medical treatments for physical system ED are limited, help can be found. For example, there are specialty clinics, often part of your state medical school, that specialize in areas such as gender dysphoria and paraphilia as well as endocrine and neurologic disorders. Oral medications (such as Cialis, Levitra, or Viagra) and other medical techniques can be helpful.

Because there is evidence that sexual orientation has roots in the biological system, it is important to personally accept your sexual orientation; changing orientation is not possible. (Consider the absurdity of trying to change a heterosexual man into a homosexual man.) Acceptance is the healthiest response. For bisexual men, adaptation may include learning to focus your sexual interests.

TREATMENTS FOR PHYSICAL ILLNESS ED

If you are concerned that a physical illness may be causing your ED, talk with your physician. Your doctor can treat the specific medical illness that has caused your ED. For example, if your doctor diagnoses a thyroid problem, he can prescribe medication to balance thyroid production; this may in turn correct your ED. Often, when the medical illness is corrected, sexual function spontaneously returns. In cases when it does not, addressing other features (for example, chemical dependency, relationship conflict, or performance anxiety) can help your recovery. Remember the fix-and-foster principle. In cases of chronic illness, ED can be effectively treated with general medical interventions and by enhancing psychological and relationship factors.

TREATMENTS FOR PHYSICAL INJURY ED

Medical treatments for the injuries that cause ED (such as spinal cord injury, stroke, or pelvic fractures) are limited. Some injuries permanently compromise the physical systems of erection and cannot be repaired. However, there are medical interventions that can bypass the impaired system or compensate for it. For example, when an injury results in permanent neurological damage, treatment with medication or a penile vacuum device may help by bypassing the damaged neurologic system.

When the medical options are not effective, sex therapy can help you learn to adapt to a permanent impairment. If you cannot "fix" the problem, you'll want to cooperate as a couple to foster your intimacy.

TREATMENT FOR LIFESTYLE ISSUES ED

Medical treatments for ED caused by an unhealthy lifestyle can be very helpful. But in this type of ED, your persistence and determination to make lifestyle changes is very important. Whether you address the issue with medical help or on your own, your resolution to achieve change is essential.

Chemical Abuse

The most common lifestyle cause of ED is alcohol consumption. Treatment is straightforward: limit your intake or stop. You can test whether your alcohol intake is a cause of your ED by abstaining from alcohol for a month to see if your erections are satisfactory. If you stop drinking and have consistent erections, you have verified that alcohol is the cause. If you cannot moderate your drinking or quit altogether, it is likely that you need to seek professional help. Drug abuse is another major factor in ED, and the same treatment suggestions apply.

Sleep Deprivation

Sustained and chronic lack of sleep can be difficult to correct, especially if you have a demanding career, family responsibilities, or both. Sleep deprivation can be caused by a medical problem. If you suspect a disorder like sleep apnea, seek a medical evaluation. Worry or anxiety is a common cause of insomnia, and addressing an underlying psychological issue may help you change the sleep deprivation pattern.

Short-term sleep medications are not usually a good option. Medications (including over-the-counter drugs) can further disrupt your sleep and exacerbate the problem. Be careful but decisive. Chronic poor sleep can affect your sexual desire as well as erections. A "low battery" is not conducive to healthy sexual functioning, let alone your general health.

Fatigue

With our hectic contemporary lifestyle, fatigue may be the most important and least obvious cause of sexual difficulties. The drain of intense work demands, commuting, parenting, social activities, and the stresses of daily living can be profound. Many couples engage in sex at the end of the day, when fatigue is at its peak. A good strategy is to be sexual in the morning, after a nap, or in the early evening, when you have the energy for an involved, satisfying sexual encounter.

Smoking

Smoking—and passive exposure to cigarette smoke—is now known to cause ED by damaging the penile vascular system (Cummins and Miller 2003). Quitting smoking is a healthy, long-term preventative move. See the Resources section at the end of this book for guidance. Your doctor, together with your partner, can help you decide on a change plan.

Poor Physical Condition and Significant Overweight

The strain on your body because of overweight or poor physical condition may impair erections, especially with aging. Your body has to work harder, and sexual function can be impaired some or all of the time. Overweight and a sedentary lifestyle with poor physical conditioning may limit the physiologic responses of arousal such as your respiration, heart capacity, and vascular efficiency. When severe, this can limit sexual response of men even in their twenties.

While the effort to overcome this cause of ED requires persistence, patience, and determination, it is something you can correct. It is best to work with the direction of your physician and a personal trainer to help you to be realistic in your change plan. It also helps enhance motivation if you work out with a "buddy"—another opportunity to work with your partner.

TREATMENT FOR DRUG SIDE-EFFECT ED

If you suspect that ED is caused by a medication you are currently taking, talk with your doctor or pharmacist about your medication dosage and options. Addressing drug side-effect ED involves (1) using strategies to circumvent or evade the unwanted sexual side effect, (2) using an additional drug (an "antidote") to counteract or offset the negative sexual side effect, or (3) compensating for ED by using a prosexual medication, such as Viagra, Levitra, or Cialis. Any medication has the potential to detrimentally affect your sexual functioning, but you should be careful not to jump to the conclusion that medication is causing your ED. Even among medications identified as potentially causing ED, only 2 to 30 percent of patients are typically affected.

Circumvention Strategies

When ED results from a medication you are taking, you and your doctor should discuss the possibility of stopping or switching to a different medication with fewer side effects if it is medically safe to do so. If normal function does not return, you should suspect additional causes of your ED. Another possibility, if medically permissible, is to take drug "holidays," brief periods without taking the medication thought to cause ED.

If your ED is caused by an antidepressant medication you have recently started taking, consider simply waiting one or two months to see if your body adjusts to the medication. Or, work with your doctor to decrease the dosage to the minimal effective dose. Sometimes you can bypass ED by scheduling sexual activity the farthest time away from the dose.

If your ED results from an antihypertensive or cardiovascular drug, your doctor can consider switching you to an ACE inhibitor such as captopril, which is less likely to cause sex dysfunction.

Medication "Antidotes"

When circumvention strategies do not work and your health requires that you continue taking the medication, taking an "antidote" may be effective. Some of the medications used to correct drug side-effect ED (especially ED caused by antidepressants) are amantadine, bethanechol, bupropion, dextroamphetamine, methylphenidate, and neostigmine (Segraves and Balon 2003). The effectiveness of these medications as an antidote varies considerably from person to person and is known to depend on dosage.

Compensation Strategies

When circumvention strategies or antidote medications are not effective, other agents such as Viagra, Levitra, or Cialis may compensate for drug side-effect ED. Men who do not want to take one of these medications or an antidote medication can consider other medical and psychological treatments.

TREATMENTS FOR ED WITH ANOTHER SEXUAL DYSFUNCTION (MIXED ED)

Mixed ED frequently involves an interaction of causes and effects, and you'll need to understand these in order to treat it effectively. For example, in about one-third of cases of ED that occurs with premature ejaculation (PE), ED is caused by overcompensation for PE, or PE is caused by overcompensation for ED (Loudon 1998). Trying to avoid ED or PE, you unwittingly induce the other dysfunction. If you have ED with PE, an oral medication such as Zoloft (sertraline) may help by relieving your performance anxiety about PE. If your ED is overcompensation for PE, our book *Coping with Premature Ejaculation* (New Harbinger Publications, 2003) may guide you to resolve the problem. Medication to ensure erections may also relieve performance anxiety and indirectly help resolve PE when it is caused by the expectation that you will have ED. In other cases, mixed ED may involve a physical problem.

Similarly, when ED occurs with low sexual desire, sexual pain, or inhibited ejaculation, it is important to address any medical cause and integrate medical treatments with psychological, relationship, and psychosexual skills interventions to resolve the multiple sexual dysfunctions. As you consider your treatment options, remember to follow our integrative principle: fix and foster.

If there are no identified physical causes, then reconsider the possibility of psychological or relationship distress. Mixed ED commonly involves a deficit in psychosexual skills, and skills learning may become your treatment of choice. Couple sex therapy may help remedy the detrimental effects of ED on you and your relationship.

ED and Your Partner's Sexual Dysfunction

When your partner has a medical or psychological problem, you may experience ED as a response. Remember that sexual function is an interpersonal process. Your sexual experience includes picking up subtle feelings from your partner. For example, her anticipation of pain due to a urinary tract or yeast infection may cause her to feel hesitant or apprehensive about sex, which can cause ED (when you then feel cautious) or PE (when you do not want to cause her physical pain). Whether your ED is caused by a physical factor in your body or indirectly by a factor in her body, the medical problem needs to be addressed and resolved. To not heal her physical or psychological problem will likely block your return to satisfying erections and lovemaking.

GENERAL MEDICAL TREATMENTS FOR ED

There are several medical treatments that are not specific to a particular type of ED but can be effective in restoring erections.

Medications for ED

Using medication is not a sign of weakness but a choice that many men find is an important resource in gaining comfort and confidence with erections. However, for some men, medication use implies the need to depend on an external resource rather than their own abilities and does not support their sexual self-esteem. Pharmacologic treatment alone is often insufficient because of the lack of response, the reluctance to consistently use prescription medications, or complicating psychological and relationship features. There are also concerns about the unknown effects of long-term use of medications.

Medication must be prescribed and monitored by a physician. Weighing the costs and the benefits of medications is part of your decision making as a couple. Obtaining the desired effect can be a matter of trial and error of different medications and dosages. New medical treatments for ED are being developed. Ask your doctor what is currently available. We strongly advise against self-medication with alcohol, recreational drugs, or over-the-counter remedies, as they have their own obvious risks.

Pro-Sex Oral Medications

Medications such as Levitra, Viagra, and Cialis help initiate and maintain erection by relaxing the corpus cavernosum smooth muscle in your penis. Viagra is the oldest of these drugs and has a longer clinical track record. Levitra similarly enhances penile blood flow with improved erections. Cialis, the newest of the three, is marketed as the "weekender" for its long-lasting results. All three medications enhance blood flow to the penis by blocking the PDE-5 enzyme. Such medications can be used for ED whether its cause is physical, psychological, or medication-related.

Yocon (yohimbine), an extract from an African tree, has been used for a number of years to aid erections by affecting the corpus cavernosum in the penis. Side effects include headache, high blood pressure, nervousness, and excitability. Most men will respond better to the more potent PDE-5 medications (Cialis, Levitra, or Viagra).

Comparing Cialis, Levitra, and Viagra

As yet there are no good scientific studies that compare the relative effectiveness and side effects of these three medications. It appears that they are approximately equal in efficacy. Effectiveness studies suggest that when you take the drug and there is adequate penile stimulation, you will have a sufficient erection for intercourse 40 to 80 percent of the time (depending on the severity of your ED).

There are some differences in the medications. For example, Viagra and Levitra work in about thirty to sixty minutes, while Cialis works in as little as thirty minutes. The erection-enhancing effect may last for approximately four hours with Viagra and four to five hours with Levitra, while Cialis' effectiveness may last for up to thirty-six hours.

Each pill sometimes (in 5-15 percent of men) produces side effects like headache, facial redness, upset stomach, back pain, and sinus congestion. The blue vision or light sensitivity some men experience with Viagra does not occur with Levitra and Cialis. Each medication has a warning about use with alpha-blocker antihypertensive (blood pressure) medications that are often used to treat enlargement of the prostate. Levitra cannot be safely taken with any alpha-blocker (e.g., Hytrin (terazosin), Flomax (tamsulosin), Cardura (doxazosin mesylate)) while for Viagra in doses above 25 mg there is a warning to stagger the dose of Viagra by 4 hours after taking an alpha-blocker. Cialis also is not to be taken with most alpha blockers, although it may be used with Flomax (0.4 mg/day) with no staggering of doses. While none of these medications has been shown to increase the risk of heart attack, the three medications cannot be taken safely with nitrates (such as Imdur (isosorbide) or nitroglycerine) for chest pain due to angina.

The choice of medication will depend upon your and your doctor's preferences. Remember that a medication's effect can vary person to person. With your doctor's supervision, try the one of your choice and adjust the dose or try another to seek the effect you want. Remember, it is crucial to integrate the medication into your couple sexual relationship.

Antianxiety Medications

Antianxiety medicines may also be useful. Medications that are effective in treating generalized anxiety and panic attacks can help some men when ED results from performance anxiety. These medications include Librium (chlordiazepoxide), Ativan (lorazepam), Valium (diaze-pam), and Xanax (alprazolam). Some of these medications can be taken as needed, one to four hours before beginning sex. However, these medications are risky, as they can be addictive. When anxiety is mild to moderate, learning anxiety management and relaxation techniques is a better choice. For sexual anxiety, learning psychosexual skills can be an effective treatment.

Medications Applied to the Penis

ED can be treated with alprostadil, a medication applied directly to the penis in one of two ways.

PGE1. The most commonly used form of alprostadil is *prostaglandin E1* (PGE1), which you inject into the base of the penis a few minutes before sexual activity. PGE1 may be used two to three times a week. When erection is assured by injection therapy, men with ED can relax and enter into an erotic flow. However, injection therapy has a high dropout rate because the man or his partner finds it awkward and clinical.

MUSE. Medicated Urethral System for Erection (MUSE) is a device used to insert an alprostadil suppository into the urethral opening. Eighty percent of the drug is absorbed after ten minutes. Reports of its effectiveness vary from 7 to 65 percent. The most common adverse effects are penile pain, urethral burning, dizziness, and fainting. MUSE also has a very high dropout rate.

Devices for ED

In addition to pharmacologic treatments, devices are sometimes used, although scientific validation of their effectiveness is limited.

Rejoyn. Nonsurgical prostheses include splints such as Rejoyn, a soft rubber brace that holds the flaccid penis rigid. The brace exposes the tip of the penis to allow for pleasure. Some women find the device uncomfortable during intercourse. These are available without prescription at many drug stores.

Vacuum Constriction Devices. Vacuum constriction devices draw blood into the penis, causing an erection, and trap the blood there in order to maintain the erection for intercourse. These devices include a plastic tube that fits over the penis to create an airtight cover. A vacuum is created around the penis by motor or manual pumping. When erection occurs, a fitted rubber band is placed on the penis at the base to retain the erection. An erection may be maintained for approximately thirty minutes. These devices require your doctor's prescription and, again, there is a high drop-out rate due to lack of comfort on the part of either the man or the woman.

Surgical Penile Prostheses

Rigid or flexible rods may be surgically implanted into the penis to make it mechanically erect. There are inflatable models that allow for artificial engorging and deflating of the penis by means of a hydraulic system composed of tubes implanted in the penis and a fluid reservoir or bulb implanted in one of the testicular sacs (the testis is removed). The tubes are then inflated by squeezing the bulb and deflated by a valve in the bulb. These surgeries do not allow for an actual erection, but they do permit the penis to be inserted into the vagina. Because implants are irreversible and do not allow any other treatments, an implant is the last option for treating ED.

Penile Vascular Surgery

When there is clearly irreversible damage to the penile arteries and veins, penile vascular reconstruction surgery may be attempted. The results of such surgery are usually poor. Such surgery is considered experimental, but its effectiveness may improve with increased medical knowledge and surgical experience.

Combination Treatments

Some physicians experiment with combination treatments that include several medications and interventions designed to overcome physical (for example, vascular or neurologic) or psychological (performance anxiety or depression) limitations. For example, Cialis combined with a vacuum device may be helpful in a severe case.

APPROACH MEDICAL TREATMENT INCREMENTALLY

In considering your medical options, think incrementally. Begin with the treatment that is the least physically intrusive and least medically risky. Certainly do not begin with an irreversible treatment, such as surgery. Remember to do all that you need to be successful, but be careful to not overdo it. To purchase a space shuttle when you only need a golf cart is excessive and involves needless risk. As long as you are comprehensive and are not missing contributing factors, you can do the least to get the most.

MEDICAL TREATMENTS HAVE LIMITATIONS

While the medical treatments we've discussed in this chapter are helpful for many men with ED, they each have limitations and rarely are effective as stand-alone treatments. They succeed best when used along with the psychosexual skills program and integrated into your flexible couple sexual style. If you expect a medical treatment to allow you erections 100 percent of the time, you subvert the 85-percent guideline of good-enough couple sexuality that establishes genuine confidence.

Your Body and Person Are Intertwined

Your body and person are intrinsically intertwined. Appreciating and respecting that your personality is fundamentally grounded or housed in your body is important. With your body healed, or the reality of its limitations understood, you are ready to pursue the psychological and relationship skills to manage your ED, enhance your intimacy, and renew sexual satisfaction.

7

Interventions for Psychological and Relationship Erectile Dysfunction

This chapter will help you address psychological system ED, psychological distress ED, relationship distress ED, mixed ED, and psychosexual skills ED. We suggest an approach to deal with psychological causes and effects, and we offer recommendations for addressing the relationship identity, cooperation, and intimacy features that may be involved with your relationship distress ED. Finally, we help you prepare for learning the psychosexual skills, especially developing positive and realistic cognitions.

APPROACHES TO RELIEVE PSYCHOLOGICALLY CAUSED ED

Let's look at ways to approach ED caused by either temporary or longstanding individual psychological distress. It's important that you be open to evaluation and treatment for chemical dependency if you have been "medicating" yourself with alcohol or drugs (see the Resources section).

Strategies to Resolve Psychological System ED

If you believe you may have psychological system ED, you can gain insight by consulting a well-respected book about the type of psychological problem you suspect, searching for psychology information and self-tests at trustworthy Internet sites, or seeking feedback from your partner or someone else you trust. Consider what you know about your family history (for example, "Grandpa was always depressed" or "Aunt Mary was obsessive about keeping the house clean") that may represent a genetic vulnerability (be "passed down").

Psychological system ED is very difficult to address with self-help approaches. An evaluation with a psychologist may help confirm your problem and help you develop a comprehensive treatment strategy. Psychologists who specialize in the area you suspect could be causing your ED—chronic depression, obsessive-compulsive disorder, phobias, bipolar disorder, generalized anxiety disorder—will be accepting and nonjudgmental.

Treatment for ED caused by a psychological system problem may include individual or group psychotherapy, medication, and sex therapy. Because your psychological problem is complex and tends to resist change, realize that it may take a considerable amount of time and effort in therapy to resolve it. When you feel ready, you can progress to learning the psychosexual skills to restore your erections.

■ James's Story: Dysthymic Depression

Thirty-two-year-old James had suffered ED all of his life and with several partners. He believed that he simply had a "dead" penis. Although he had full erections when he awoke, he usually masturbated with 75 percent erection or less. He was not able to have an erection or ejaculate with a partner, however. He thought he was a failure as a man and told himself so constantly.

James asked his physician what could cause him to have a "little" penis. The doctor examined his genitals and found him normal. It was another two years before James found the courage to again ask about his "little" penis and how he could "make it bigger." This time the doctor was attentive enough to ask exactly what he was concerned about, and James explained that his penis was "never full." James was referred to a urologist for a thorough evaluation involving physical exam, penile blood pressure, and arterial testing with injection evaluation and sonography. All of James's tests were in the normal range. His physical body was fine.

James and his physician ruled out physiological causes, and he was referred to a psychologist who specialized in sex therapy to consider a psychological cause. Through his interview and psychological testing, the psychologist determined that James was burdened with dysthymia, or chronic, persistent depression. The therapist believed that this was the basis for James's ED. It also became clear that James felt a significant amount of shame about being a sexual man, believing his sexual desires (even though appropriate for an adult male) to be immoral. In individual psychotherapy, he addressed his dysthymia as well as the sexual shame. An antidepressant medication helped to lift the cloud that James felt was "parked" over him. His physician selected Wellbutrin because of its limited sexual side effects. With psychotherapy, medication to alleviate his depression, and psychosexual skills training, James learned to relax his body and focus on the pleasure. As he gained better erections, his confidence increased.

Strategies to Resolve Individual Psychological Distress ED

If you believe you have psychological distress ED, review what you noted to be the stressors, and explore other types of ED that might be causing psychological distress that worsens your sexual problem. Most men prefer to address the specific psychological stressor using self-help efforts, since this type of problem is less severe and chronic than psychological system ED.

Among your options, consider reading a reliable book or visiting a reputable Web site on the type of stress you suspect (such as depression, anxiety, grieving) and how to adapt (see Resources). If reading and reflecting is not your style, or if your self-help approach is not effective, use good judgment and seek professional therapy. The clinician can help you gain perspective, offer objective psychological testing, and help you consider strategies for change. If marital issues are causing your psychological distress (for example, an affair has led to depression), this needs to be addressed in couple therapy. Medication may be beneficial in addressing depression or anxiety rooted in current stresses.

Men tend to minimize or downplay their psychological upset and anguish—a very common and self-defeating coping strategy. Men try to "tough it out" and divert attention. This emotional avoidance does not resolve the psychological distress and becomes a barrier to emotional intimacy. It may be difficult for you to appreciate that distressing personal feelings can cause or maintain ED. While most daily stresses can be handled by "moving on," some important issues can't be avoided without causing further psychological and sexual problems. Unless you are having significant relationship conflict, consider sharing your feelings with your intimate partner so she has the opportunity to be your primary support. In some cases, resolution of the psychological problem will restore healthy sexual function, while in others the psychosexual skill exercises or coaching with a sex therapist may be needed to overcome problems such as anticipatory anxiety, performance anxiety, or loss of sexual confidence. These features can maintain your ED even when the original cause has been resolved.

When Your Partner Is Psychologically Distressed

Your partner's psychological distress can cause ED by negatively affecting your relationship. When you feel her tension during lovemaking, your body reflexively responds with tentativeness or diminished sexual desire. Even when it is mild, your partner's distress can subvert your sexual function.

In dealing with her psychological distress, your empathy and emotional support is important. This is an opportunity to build deeper intimacy by cooperatively addressing the problem.

APPROACHES TO ALLEVIATE RELATIONSHIP DISTRESS ED

If you feel you have relationship distress ED, focus on the interpersonal dynamics you believe might be causing, maintaining, or resulting from your ED. You can heal the harm by addressing the most common cognitive, behavioral, and emotional features of your relationship distress. The Resources section lists books you may find helpful in resolving relationship distress.

Your Partner's Dissatisfaction

Even though you may feel satisfied with your relationship except for the ED, your partner may feel lonely or disconnected and long for more emotional intimacy. Your partner's dissatisfaction may be a factor in causing your ED as well as a result of it. Don't stick your head in the sand; ask her how she feels. You may wish to avoid dealing with her disappointment, but addressing this is necessary to resolve your ED.

Addressing Relationship Distress

The CBE model, which we introduced in chapter 4, can guide your approach to alleviate relationship distress. You will need to work on one or more of the following objectives:

Identity: Clarifying and integrating your relationship and sexual cognitions, balancing individual autonomy and your couple bonding.

Cooperation: Modifying your interpersonal behaviors to address problems such as communication deficits or a conflict-resolution impasse.

Intimacy: Enhancing your emotional empathy in order to heal relationship injuries and promote emotional alliance.

■ Todd and Jennifer

Todd and Jennifer were troubled. He worked as a teacher and she as a financial analyst for a large financial institution. They were busy with two children, ages two and four. Jennifer felt irritated and slighted that Todd acted as though his career was more important than hers, and that he religiously played soccer with his buddies every Tuesday evening and then socialized until late at the local sports bar. He felt unappreciated, arguing that he worked hard to provide for his family and spent as much time as he could with the children. He encouraged her to have a night out with her girlfriends, but she declined, claiming she had no time and no energy.

The frustrations came to the surface one evening when they argued bitterly about his evening out with the guys. She accused him of abandoning her, caring more for his buddies than for her. Todd felt falsely accused and angrily accused her of being impossible to please, always complaining and demanding. The argument ended in silence and avoidance.

Several weeks later, when Todd could not keep his erection during lovemaking, tensions erupted again. In her frustration, Jennifer abruptly said, "If you can't keep it up, stop pestering me with sex! You don't do anything to help out with the kids, and I am too tired for sex anyway!" Stunned, he shot back that she caused his erection problem by being a sexual turnoff. Thereafter, sexual frequency dramatically declined, and ED became their common experience. Each avoided talking, afraid things would become even more hostile.

What began as a very common relationship issue—balancing individual autonomy with relationship cohesion—got out of hand and precipitated personal, relationship, and sexual dysfunction. Conflict over balancing individuality and relationship cohesion (defining relationship identity) led to arguing, criticism, and avoidance rather than cooperation for mutual conflict resolution. This cooperation deficit left each feeling frustrated and victimized. For Todd and Jennifer, resolving ED required attention to the individual and relationship distress which both caused and maintained ED.

Improving Your Relationship Identity

Your cognitions (beliefs, assumptions, perceptions, attributions, and expectations) about yourself, your partner, and how to be a couple make up your relationship identity. Your cognitions about sexuality and being intimate partners compose your sexual identity. Differences and misunderstandings are normal and expected. Clarifying misunderstandings and integrating healthier understandings into your couple style is part of reducing relationship distress. This forms the foundation for cooperation and intimacy.

EXERCISE: Clarifying Your Relationship Identity

Consider your thoughts and feelings about how well you balance individuality and relationship cohesion. First, answer the following questions individually. Then, talk with your partner about what you believe a relationship should involve and how to "do" a satisfying relationship.

1. What are your expectations about how to communicate, deal with conflicts, express affection?

2. What do you each believe and feel about gender roles, the importance of sex, your parents as a marital and sexual model, prior relationship experiences, spiritual beliefs, career goals, friendships, loyalties, and leisure and social activities?

3. What do you bring to your relationship? Leadership, kindness, energy, calmness, optimism, emotion, reason, warmth, work ethic, commitment to family, playfulness and humor? What do you feel proud of? What does your partner bring to the relationship that you appreciate?

4. What expectations do you have for your relationship, and how well are these being met?

5. How highly do you and your partner prioritize your relationship? How important is your partner to you? You to your partner? Do you have sufficient time together?

6. To what degree do you approach daily life with a team mentality?

7. How do you feel about the amount of autonomy in your marriage? Do you feel as independent as you want? Free or constrained? Do you have your own activities, interests? Do you have as much time for yourself as you need? Where is your place to be alone, "off duty"?

Balance in your relationship identity is the environment in which cooperation can thrive.

Improving Your Relationship Cooperation

Cooperation provides a safe environment for learning psychosexual skills and gives each partner the opportunity to heal from old hurts and frustrations.

Conflict Is Your Opportunity for Intimacy

While many couples view disagreements as a threat to their intimacy, in truth, addressing conflict is the ordinary, day-to-day process through which you can deepen your intimacy. When you have a dispute with the goal of prevailing in what you want, your partner feels unimportant, disregarded, and rejected. However, when you bring a spirit of cooperation and mutual empathy, you can learn to understand the meaning and deeper feelings behind the conflict. You can participate in finding a mutually satisfying resolution.

Resolving Conflict Mutually

To mutually resolve conflicts, especially conflicts about ED, you need to be vulnerable and invest your thoughts and feelings. This requires communicating as friends, not adversaries. Frame your issue as a couple problem. Ask yourselves, "How do *we* resolve *our* problem in such a way that *we* both feel good about it?" This includes addressing ED as "our" problem.

The great majority of mutual solutions are *mosaic* solutions, meaning that they are made up of several ideas and behaviors which each partner contributes to a resolution. Avoid either-or solutions, which create a winner and loser. *The guiding principle for effective conflict resolution is that each partner feels emotionally satisfied with the outcome.*

Win-win solutions are not always achievable. When this is the reality, you need to accept your differences. Most couples are capable of doing this when they feel a sense of equity and both are willing to compromise. *Toleration* of disparity is adequate; *acceptance* of differences is satisfying; and *integration* of diversity is ideal.

EXERCISE: Evaluating Your Cooperation

Do you feel your partner is demanding? How competitive are you in the relationship? Do you have destructive arguments? Do your disagreements leave lasting hurt? Have you offered forgiveness of each other (and yourself) for the hurts? Can you be patient, warm, and kind with your partner? Are the outcomes to your disagreements emotionally satisfying for each? Are you ready to cooperate to do the skills training and improve your sexual life?

Improving Your Emotional Intimacy

The most important goal and predictor of success—and the greatest reward—is relationship intimacy. Your relationship is the "system" or environment for mutual support, acceptance, and empathy. Have you been afraid of deeper intimacy and solid closeness? Are there hidden hurts that linger? Are you holding a grudge?

Empathy requires forgiving yourself and your partner for past hurts and disappointments—no matter how small or how monumental. If you do not forgive, resentment will block cooperation and interfere with your capacity to relax your body, focus on pleasurable sensations, and learn psychosexual skills. The future will feel different if you acknowledge the past and forgive yourself and each other. You each need to focus on promoting your partner's emotional satisfaction.

Identity, Cooperation, and Intimacy in Your Sexual Relationship

ED exists within a relationship, not in a vacuum. Being an intimate team requires you to understand and accept each other as sexual partners. The following exercise will help you discuss the identity, cooperation, and intimacy dimensions of your sexual relationship. Understanding each other enhances cooperation with lovemaking and allows you to feel pleasure and closeness.

EXERCISE: Clarifying Your Sexual Relationship Identity

Discuss your thoughts about the following dimensions of your sexual relationship:

1. How openly can you talk of your sexual wants, dislikes, joys, comfort, ideas? Is there anything about your sexuality that you do not want to discuss?

2. To what extent might differences about the balance of autonomy and relationship cohesion be an irritant that you bring into the bedroom?

3. What does it mean to balance individuality and coupleness during sex? Is individuality selfish? Does cohesion seem confining or smothering?

4. Does your sex have to be either intense, raw, and passionate or deeply personal and romantic?

5. What does sex mean to you? What role should sex play in your relationship? A source of emotional vitality? Procreation? Pleasure? Duty? Joy? Passion? Tension release? Harmony? Romance?

6. What are you proud of sexually? What does your partner bring to the sexual relationship that you appreciate? What percent of your lovemaking do you think should be fantastic, and what makes it

fantastic? What percent should be satisfying? What percent okay? What percent poor quality, and what makes it so?

7. How do you feel about lovemaking where you take turns pleasing each other compared to mutually, simultaneously making love? Do you and your partner expect to take turns being "sexually selfish?"

8. Do you agree that there is more than one kind of sex? (Quickies? Impulsive passion? Mechanical anxiety release? Romance?)

9. Do you expect sexual pleasure to decrease or increase over time? Why do you think this? Do you believe sex can improve?

10. Can you be sexually playful? Tender? Can sex bring consolation during stressful periods? Do you share the standard of good-enough sex?

Share your thoughts. Your sexual relationship identity is founded upon who each of you is as a unique individual and what you bring to your sex life.

ED and Sexual Relationship Cooperation

Relationship cooperation is essential to being an intimate team. How well do you work together to give and receive sensual pleasure? Do you care for each other's wishes and desires? How well can you pursue mutual pleasure rather than individual performance?

ED and Sexual Intimacy

In the emotional life of your relationship, ED can bring about hurtful feelings (humiliation, rejection, loneliness, failure, or abandonment) that undermine positive feelings (acceptance, closeness, and love). The emotional suffering of couples with ED is quiet, hidden, and often deeply upsetting, which only adds to the confusion and sense of hopelessness. The first step to recover from the emotional distress of ED is to verbally forgive yourself and your partner for the past sexual hurt, disappointment, and alienation. Do not hold yourself and each other emotionally hostage for the past. Forgiveness facilitates working as a team to overcome your ED. Keep your perspective. Relationship intimacy is your ultimate goal and your ultimate reward.

APPROACHES TO ALLEVIATE PSYCHOSEXUAL SKILLS ED

If you believe your ED is caused primarily by a deficit in psychosexual skills, you will certainly need to build those skills in order to overcome ED. But regardless of the cause of your ED, you and your partner can benefit tremendously from improving your psychosexual skills.

The Four Ps for Sexual Skills Development

A skill, whether cognitive, emotional, behavioral, or interpersonal, is the learned ability to perform the task well and with some ease. Skills are developed and enriched through the four Ps: practice, persistence, patience, and partnership.

If you worry that our change program will be too difficult, reassure yourself that these skills are very manageable because you do them in increments. Practice and repetition makes them easier. You might not feel optimistic because your past efforts brought no real success. Don't give up. Your fear that our comprehensive approach might not work is understandable; you have no reason to believe you will succeed. It is okay to be skeptical. Then, when you begin to make progress, you will be pleased. This is not to encourage you to be pessimistic, but rather to remind you that you can't force the change you seek. Loosen up, be persistent, and let our approach prove itself. Optimism and satisfaction is the caboose on the train. Wait for it. Your efforts, step-by-step, will pay off with wonderful feelings of satisfaction with yourself, your partner, and your lovemaking. Yes, learning these skills is an effort; there is no easy fix. But enjoying arousal, erections, and couple sexuality is worth it.

Cognitive Preparation for Your Psychosexual Skills Work

The most important sex organ in your body is your mind. Prepare yourself mentally to engage in the change process.

Think about Sex in Terms of Pleasure

People engage in couple sex for multiple reasons:

- for reproduction, the "natural" or biological function of sex;

- for physical and sensual pleasure, a prime motivator;

- as a tension release to ease the stresses of everyday living;

- to increase your self-esteem and self-worth; and

- to foster as well as celebrate love, affection, delight, closeness, and couple fulfillment.

In healthy relationships, sex has multiple positive purposes. But when sex becomes one-dimensional (for example, to prove your erectile performance), you set yourself up for ED. Sex as a pass-fail performance interferes with the positive functions of sexuality, bringing distress to both you and your partner. As long as you focus solely on performance, you will suffer performance anxiety that exacerbates and reinforces ED. *If you are to resolve ED, you must think about sex in terms of pleasure, self-esteem, and intimacy as well as good-enough erections.*

Integrate the Styles of Sexual Arousal

Your mental focus is the essential feature of sexual arousal (Mosher 1980). Men with ED invariably and exclusively use arousal strategies that focus on their partner (her body, her responses, and the "sexy" or "romantic" interaction) or on erotic fantasy. They also tend to constantly monitor their erection. This focus exclusively on the partner is called *partner interaction arousal,* while monitoring your erection is called *spectatoring.* Both strategies divert attention from your body and your own sensual experience and diminish your ability to obtain and maintain an erection. You will need to learn another type of sexual arousal, *sensual self-entrancement,* which involves focusing your attention primarily on your body, on your own physical sensations and sensual pleasure. This type of arousal promotes relaxation and eliminates spectatoring. Gradually, you will blend and balance both sensual self-entrancement and partner interaction arousal to enjoy confident erections and satisfying sex.

Take Responsibility for Your Sexual Growth

Part of mental preparedness is establishing a clear, positive attitude toward sex; realistic expectations; and a deep commitment to mutual sexual satisfaction. Take personal responsibility for pursuing your sexual growth. Being responsible means intentionally engaging in the change steps, even when they may seem counterintuitive.

Changing the Way You Think about Sex

Your cognitions make up the sexual "meaning" of ED. These cognitions influence your emotional experiences and behaviors during sex. For example, if you think you are a failure or a wimp, you will feel defeated, depressed, and inferior and act frustrated or angry. Or, if you think sex is bad, you will feel shame and disgust and likely act by withdrawing or avoiding sex. On the other hand, if you think of your sexual interactions as cooperative, healthy, playful, and mutually pleasurable, you will feel confidence, comfort, closeness, and satisfaction. Affirm that sex is good. Pleasure is good. Sharing your body with your lover is good.

The meaning of ED has substantial emotional significance. When the meaning of ED is hidden for you and your partner, or when you are reluctant or unable to discuss the meaning that ED has for you, it is difficult to share the change experience and cooperate. Identifying and understanding the meaning of ED provides an important foundation for you to accept your dilemma and begin to replace detrimental cognitions, actions, and feelings with beneficial ones. Addressing ED as a couple will help you develop new sexual and relationship meanings, a crucial resource in overcoming ED. Dealing with ED is an opportunity to deepen relationship intimacy.

EXERCISE: Replacing Your Negative ED Cognitions

There are a number of detrimental thoughts that may cause, maintain, or exacerbate your ED. Review the examples below. Our coaching comments help you understand how such thoughts are detrimental, and the sample replacement offers a beneficial alternative. Create your own replacement thoughts to correct your detrimental thoughts and develop more realistic and reasonable cognitions. Write out these beneficial replacement thoughts so you can remember them later.

Detrimental belief: *There is nothing worse in a sexual relationship than losing your erection. ED is a train wreck.*

Coaching comment: No man wants to have ED, but remember that a simplistic focus on sex performance rather than a focus on pleasure and couple cooperation is the real train wreck.

Sample replacement: *When I lose my erection, it is an opportunity for cooperation and emotional intimacy.*

Your beneficial replacement:

Detrimental belief: *Erections should be automatic and happen when I have the opportunity, when I want one, and for as long as I want.*

Coaching comment: Are you sure you want to think of yourself as a sex machine rather than a real man? Do you really believe that your partner wants a sex robot more than a man? Talk with her about this.

Sample replacement: *I am not a machine. My penis is human. I will be realistic in my sexual expectations.*

Your beneficial replacement:

Detrimental belief: *When I lose my erection, I disappoint the very woman I love. I must apologize, withdraw, and go away because I am a complete failure.*

Coaching comment: Your sensitivity to your partner's feelings is good, but your reaction is detrimental. Apologizing, withdrawing, blaming yourself, and putting yourself down block couple cooperation. Stay present and be an intimate team.

Sample replacement: *When I lose my erection, I can adapt and cooperate for mutual pleasure.*

Your beneficial replacement:

Detrimental belief: *I don't really want to have sex now, but I can't ask for a rain check because I am supposed to want sex anytime.*

Coaching comment: This belief is pure pressure, which will itself cause ED. Sex on demand is unreasonable. Don't set yourself up to fail with this performance pressure.

Sample replacement: *I can ask for a rain check or let her know I want to give her what she'd like by touch this time.*

Your beneficial replacement:

Detrimental belief: *If I can't get or keep my erection, I am a wimp.*

Coaching comment: ED does not make you a wimp. Denigrating yourself is self-defeating. Not cooperating with your partner for mutually satisfying sex is self-defeating. A genuine man cooperates and treats the woman as his intimate friend.

Sample replacement: *I am a good man, not a performance machine. Erect or not, I can be a caring lover.*

Your beneficial replacement:

Detrimental attribution: *She's not helping, and she seems disappointed. It's really her fault that I can't get it up or keep it up.*

Coaching comment: Be careful to not blame her for your frustration about your ED. No problem is ever fixed by blame. Erections are your responsibility. If you are not getting what you want, ask for it. If that leads to conflict, talk with her as a friend—outside the bedroom—about cooperation.

Sample replacement: *I will ask her for what I want to help relax my body and promote my erection.*

Your beneficial replacement:

Detrimental expectation: *If we try to have sex, it won't work because I'll have ED. It will be a disappointment, and she'll be angry.*

Coaching comment: Most women become "angry" (hurt) because the man gets upset with himself or blames her, and the lovemaking stops. Her reaction is more about feeling abandoned emotionally than about your sex performance. Remember: Sensual pleasure is the essence of sexuality.

Sample replacement: *If I lose my erection, I'll pleasure her with touch, and we'll be fine.*

Your beneficial replacement:

EXERCISE: Your Partner's Cognitions about ED

There are common detrimental thoughts your partner may have had, so invite her to consider the following cognitive exercise.

Detrimental belief: *Sex should always be romantic.*

Coaching comment: Normal sex may be special 10 to 20 percent of the time, pleasurable 30 to 40 percent; routine 10 to 20 percent, mediocre 10 to 20 percent, and poor 5 to 15 percent of the time.

Sample replacement: *Sex can be special, emotional, physical, romantic, routine, or even poor; it will vary from time to time.*

Beneficial replacement:

Detrimental assumption: *I am the woman; I am supposed to make him get an erection.*

Coaching comment: As satisfying as it may feel to believe that you alone cause his erection, in fact, you are the catalyst for partner interaction arousal. He can bring about his own erection by relaxing his body and managing his arousal.

Sample replacement: *He loves me, and I can be helpful by relaxing, participating, and enjoying our touch.*

Beneficial replacement:

Detrimental attribution: *He loses his erection because he does not find me attractive. It is my fault because I am not sexy enough to get and keep him hard, and I don't know what to do!*

Coaching comment: This says more about your fears of inadequacy than reality. Erection is his responsibility. Remember, your role is supportive. If you blame yourself, you will find it difficult to be an intimate team. Tell him you want to work together for mutual pleasure and intimacy.

Sample replacement: *Physical relaxation and sensual pleasure cause erections. I can help, but I can't make it happen. Only he can. Let me try to help.*

Beneficial replacement:

Practice your beneficial replacement thoughts by reading them out loud ten times to each other. You may feel silly, but the repetition will help you become more comfortable with these thoughts. Speaking them can enhance your comfort.

The Vital Cognition: Good-Enough Sex

The most important cognition for a healthy sexual relationship is that you and your partner will be most satisfied with good-enough sex. Good-enough sex is grounded in reasonable expectations of your bodies, receptivity to male and female sexual arousal, and valuing pleasure more than performance. Judging the quality of sex by performance standards like, "I must have an erection for great sex," trivializes the human value of sexual intimacy. Such perfectionism undermines the relaxation necessary for satisfying sex. Each person feeling accepted (no matter what is going on with lubrication, erections, or orgasm) is good-enough sex.

Changing the Way You Act about Sex

To address ED, you and your partner must focus on cooperative behavior that moves you toward your goal. When your ED is not constructively addressed, it manifests in negative behavior. For example, you forego sex to avoid disappointment, avoid talking about the problem, act as though nothing is wrong, pressure your partner to have orgasm to compensate for ED, or make love rigidly and mechanically as you try desperately to get or keep an erection. She may push you away, say hurtful things, rush sex to get it over with to avoid further hurt and frustration, or place limitations or conditions on sex.

ED is an opportunity for you to deepen your emotional and sexual intimacy. Differences or disagreements about sexual interaction are common and normal; the issue is how well you deal with these. ED is an example of a relationship cooperation challenge. With a positive, respectful, affirming process of conflict resolution, you develop a deeper understanding of how the other thinks and feels; a greater sense of self-esteem, respect, and admiration for each other; confidence that future conflict can be resolved; and increased goodwill and comfort, which facilitates sexual desire.

Detrimental behaviors cause, maintain, or worsen ED. You need to replace them with beneficial behaviors.

Detrimental Behaviors	Beneficial Behaviors
Profusely apologizing for losing your erection and frustrating her.	Acknowledging your penis is on "break" and inviting her to guide you to pleasure her in ways other than intercourse.
Refusing to discuss the sexual problem or withdrawing.	Talking calmly, being present, sharing your feelings, describing the dilemma you face, and asking for cooperation to enrich your sexual relationship.
Expressing frustration at yourself and your partner.	Reminding yourself that expressing frustration doesn't help, then refocusing and recommitting to enhancing sensual and sexual pleasure.
Anticipating sexual "failure" and then avoiding initiating sex.	Openly acknowledging the dilemma you feel, agreeing to maintain a regular rhythm of sexual connection, and actively engaging in affectionate, sensual, playful, and erotic touching.
Verbally criticizing your partner or your partner's behavior.	Calmly and openly expressing your own feelings.
Having sex with someone else to "test" your erections.	Expressing to your partner your desire to cooperate to resolve your ED. An affair is truly poisonous for your intimate relationship.

Changing the Way You Feel about Sex

Negative feelings about yourself because of ED can change. By positively changing the way you think about yourself as a sexual person and learning to change how you behave, you will come to feel better about yourself, your partner, and your sexual life. The way you think and what you do influence how you feel. To change emotionally, you need to develop beneficial thoughts and accept your honest feelings about ED—the discouragement, hurt, frustration, anger, apprehension, embarrassment, shame, depression. These feelings remind you that you are not satisfied with the way things are. It's time to change. Accepting your negative emotional experience allows you to stop fighting yourself. Acceptance is an important part of learning to relax during sex.

Sharing Feelings about ED

,It is important that you distinguish your feelings from your behaviors. It is healthy to be aware of your emotions (feelings) and to share them in an open, calm, and constructive manner (behavior). But understand that you do not have to engage in the behavior of *expressing* impulsive, raw negative feelings—especially frustration, irritability, or disappointment. Recognize that there are risks and harm in expressing unbridled negative emotions. Definitely refrain from expression of feelings that might be destructive during the exercises in this book. Instead, internally soothe these feelings and remember that you will learn positive feelings through new cognitions and behaviors. Expressing negative feelings will only trap you in the past and will be very discouraging for you both. If you cannot manage your negative feelings during the exercises, this is an indication that you would benefit from marital or sex therapy.

Identifying and Positively Sharing Your Feelings

Perhaps, like many men, you believe that sharing your vulnerability and revealing your deeper feelings will cause you to feel ashamed or weak. In fact, sharing feelings is a healthy part of intimacy.

To identify your feelings, you'll need to seek them out. When you focus exclusively on your thoughts (interpretations), you will concentrate on issues such as fairness or accuracy. If you focus on behaviors, then judgment of right or wrong is the focus. When you focus on feelings, you focus on the quality of what you are experiencing.

Your emotional goal is to transform detrimental feelings into constructive and beneficial ones: confidence, trust, comfort, closeness, warmth, mutual acceptance, pleasure, playfulness, collaboration. Changing your cognitions and behaviors about ED will help transform your feelings and help you enjoy good-enough sex.

Change is a process that you accomplish step by step. By preparing yourself cognitively, emotionally, behaviorally, and interpersonally, you position yourself to succeed. Practice, be patient, persist, and work as a partnership. Don't lie to yourself: This is hard work. But good things are built by effort. Do not pressure yourselves to be perfect, because this interferes with relaxing your mind and body. Follow the principle of being good enough. You *will* regain your comfort and confidence with erections and couple sexuality.

8

Psychosexual Skills: Cooperation for Pleasure

In this chapter, you will learn the psychosexual skills to obtain and maintain an erection sufficient for intercourse. We will guide you through detailed exercises to not only regain confidence with erections but also enhance desire, pleasure, arousal, and intercourse. As you learn these skills, keep your relationship perspective. Don't lose sight of the big picture. Closeness and satisfaction are the ultimate goal. Follow the four Ps of success: practice, persistence, patience, and partnership.

THE FOUR PHASES OF SKILLS LEARNING

Let's begin by giving you an overview of the skills so you understand clearly what you are trying to achieve, how each skill relates to the others, and how to put the skills together for a satisfying sexual experience. There are four phases, and this chapter will guide you through the first three phases, composed of ten steps. Chapters 9 and 10 will guide you through phase four, developing a couple sexual style and preventing relapse.

The first phase involves a series of exercises to promote physical relaxation and comfort with your sexuality. You will learn cognitive and behavioral skills for relaxing your body, which sets the foundation for pleasure and reliable erections. In step one, you'll develop ease and comfort talking about sexuality. In step two, you'll learn physical relaxation. Step three teaches you to identify and consciously use your pelvic muscle for relaxation.

The second phase offers a series of exercises to lead you to experience easy, relaxed, dependable erections. You will understand how to get an erection and build your confidence with erections. You'll develop an understanding of how to build your "erotic flow." Step four offers you a couple pleasuring exercise in which you'll enjoy relaxed, sensual touch. In step five, you will develop awareness of the range of your sexual arousal and build your cognitive erotic continuum. In step six, you'll learn more about your own genital sensations and your partner's. Step seven guides you through an exercise that shows you how to get, choose to lose, then regain erections.

The third phase involves a series of exercises to help you enjoy intercourse with new sexual confidence, pleasure, and closeness and build flexible sexual scenarios. In step eight, you will be able to integrate these skills, initiate intercourse, and become confident with erections during intercourse. In step nine, we'll guide you to calmly enjoy intercourse, encourage your partner's pleasure, and develop alternative nonintercourse scenarios. Finally, in step ten, we'll help you explore sexual variety and erotic playfulness.

GUIDELINES FOR LEARNING PSYCHOSEXUAL SKILLS

You'll want to follow some basic guidelines as you learn the skills in this chapter.

Tailor Your Steps to Your Level of Severity

Choose your approach according to the severity of your ED, which you determined in chapter 5. Work with your partner to decide what steps best fit your situation. If you are recovering from ED caused by a medical, psychological, or relationship problem (and the problem has been treated) or your problem is mild (EDSI less than forty), discuss whether you want to do all the steps or only those that you think will be relevant and helpful.

If you have moderate ED (EDSI forty to fifty-nine), completing most of the ten steps will probably be necessary to resolve your ED. Only skip those areas where you already have good-enough comfort and skill. If your program plan does not bring about the results you want, you can retrace your steps and complete them all, or you can consult a sex therapist.

If your EDSI score is severe (greater than sixty), you will need to complete every exercise. The more severe your ED, the more likely working with a marital and sex therapist would be helpful.

Do the Steps in Order

The exercises should be done in order. Working ahead or skipping steps can be risky. We know, you want to get to the good stuff, but patience is your friend. Moving too quickly will undermine your ability to relax, which is essential to progress. Take one step and one exercise at a time.

Understand the Requirements for Erections

From your body's perspective, two things are required for an erection: sufficient physiological relaxation and sufficient physical stimulation to your penis. These are related by way of an integrated exchange: The more physically relaxed you are, the less physical stimulation is required for an erection. On the other hand, the more tense or anxious you are, the more stimulation is needed. The guideline to ensure functional erections is this: *Integrate your level of physical relaxation with a graduated level of stimulation.*

Integrate the Styles of Sexual Arousal

In a healthy relationship, familiarity creates a balance, a more relaxed sexual interaction, and shifts arousal style from partner interaction arousal to sensual self-entrancement arousal. If this subtle shift does not occur, you find yourself compensating for a mellowing of sexual excitement by anxiously pursuing new forms of partner interaction arousal. Sometimes this pursuit of variety can promote excesses that stress your relationship: pressing your partner to wear new lingerie, using distasteful pornography, or even going to strip bars or having an affair. The problem develops when you fail to learn the more reliable sensual self-entrancement arousal and instead compulsively seek externally focused stimulation.

Initially, the exercises focus on sensual self-entrancement arousal; then they integrate partner interaction arousal. You'll blend the two styles of arousal for dependable erections.

What If You Experience Distress during an Exercise?

Because you're trying to extend your comfort and skill level, some exercises may cause anxiety. This is to be expected. However, should the exercise cause significant distress or discouragement (which is the opposite of what we want for you), be wise and seek professional coaching or therapy.

■ Troy and Rebecca

As you engage in the steps, Troy and Rebecca will be your guides. They learned a reasonable way of thinking about ED and a realistic approach to resolving the problem and enhancing couple sexuality, and you can too.

Troy, thirty-six, and Rebecca, thirty-five, married for nine years, by choice had no children. Each was highly invested in a demanding career, he as an insurance broker, she as an attorney. They thought their marriage to be normal; the only bumps in the road were infrequent but intense arguments about relationships with each other's parents and their social life. Four years into their marriage, Troy experienced erratic ED. He would do fine, then not, which they attributed to incidental stresses. When his ED became more common (occurring four out of five times), Troy became frustrated and expressed this by cursing and withdrawing. Rebecca lost patience with this because it ended their lovemaking. She suggested that they get help; Troy responded by withdrawing further, avoiding all discussion. He felt perplexed and sad.

Finally, he talked with his family physician about the ED, telling him that he thought it could be caused by his growing discouragement with his career or something wrong with his body. Finding no physical problems, the doctor offered him the choice of an antidepressant to relieve the distress about his career stagnation or Cialis to fix his ED. Troy responded that he was "too young" for Cialis and didn't want an antidepressant either, preferring to "tough it out." Troy wanted to regain erections without a "crutch." When things did not change, however, he finally called the psychologist his doctor recommended.

Dr. Sawyer encouraged Troy to include Rebecca in the therapy, saying that sexual problems are an intimate relationship opportunity. Together with

Dr. Sawyer, Troy and Rebecca identified that Troy's ED was caused by psychological distress from ongoing depressive feelings regarding his stagnant career, maintained by relationship distress from unresolved conflict and reinforced by Troy's uncertainty about how to deal with his body (and with Rebecca) to ensure sexual function.

Dr. Sawyer helped Troy and Rebecca address each facet of ED. Having believed that sex should be automatic and spontaneous, Troy was challenged by the amount of discipline required, but he gradually began to experience success. Rebecca especially enjoyed the sensual exercises, which felt like a more genuine, meaningful connection with Troy. Working together helped them to feel closer as a couple. During the process, if either became confused or discouraged, they reminded each other of the larger goal: relationship closeness.

Dr. Sawyer encouraged Troy and Rebecca to acknowledge that learning psychosexual skills was challenging and difficult. At first, the exercises seemed a huge intrusion into lovemaking. They came to accept this, reminding themselves that they would eventually develop a more personalized couple sexual style. Troy found that physical relaxation was the essential strategy.

Dr. Sawyer told Troy and Rebecca that when an exercise felt awkward, they could simply ignore this, instead focus on the physical sensations, and wait until after they completed the exercise to discuss their perceptions. Dr. Sawyer suggested that Troy and Rebecca thank each other after each session, no matter how poorly it might have gone. The guideline: Deeply appreciate your partner's effort, and say so.

PHASE ONE: DEVELOPING RELAXATION AND COMFORT

The exercises in phase one help increase your sexual self-esteem, teach you fundamental body management skills, and enhance your sexual comfort by inviting you to share sexual feelings. Learning relaxation will provide the foundation for later steps and help counter the performance anxiety that accompanies ED. If your body can't relax during sex, you won't obtain sufficient and enduring erections.

Step One: Increasing Sexual Comfort

Goal: Develop tranquility and assurance with your partner.

Sexual comfort feels good and creates an atmosphere in which you can successfully learn these skills. It was essential for Troy and Rebecca to know that they could express their sexual thoughts and feelings and be met with acceptance, respect, and caring. Some couples with ED avoid talking of their sexual wants out of fear it will add to performance pressure. You can develop increased sexual comfort by talking gently and openly about your positive sexual thoughts, feelings, wishes, and desires as well as your sexual discomforts, shynesses, and inhibitions. Sexual feelings are deeply personal and significant; they deserve respect and tender care.

COUPLE EXERCISE: Talking about Sexual Feelings

With mutual acceptance, share your sexual thoughts and feelings. Discuss what you learned about sexuality as a child and adolescent. What did you learn about masturbation, marriage, petting, intercourse, oral sex, orgasm, how a man and woman were supposed to act during sex? Who taught you this? What did it mean to you at the time? What does it mean to you now?

What are your attitudes and beliefs about sexuality? What is okay and what is not okay during lovemaking? What do you *believe* is okay but not *feel* is okay? What do you believe about intercourse? Oral sex? Experimentation? Sharing sexual fantasies? What do you believe about masturbating privately? Stimulating yourself while your partner watches? Mutual manual stimulation (simultaneously or taking turns)? Tell your partner what you sexually like and appreciate about her. What do you really like about couple sex? Discuss the sexual concerns you have, remembering to speak empathically, warmly, and respectfully.

Troy and Rebecca found that these open discussions facilitated their comfort. However, Troy worried that because this openness and acceptance made him feel more sexually attracted to Rebecca, ED would be an even greater disappointment. Dr. Sawyer reassured Troy that feeling this attraction was healthy.

Step Two: Training Your Mind and Body for Relaxation

Goal: Learn relaxation, the foundation for pleasure and erections.

Satisfying sexual function depends on physical relaxation. You can't duck or bypass this skill. We'll teach you to relax *in your body,* as opposed to the more common out-of-body relaxation strategies that focus on calm images (natural beauty) or soothing sounds (ocean waves). In-body relaxation helps you reduce performance anxiety and focus on the physical sensations of pleasure. Body-focused relaxation is the foundation for sensual self-entrancement arousal.

INDIVIDUAL EXERCISE: Deep Breathing

Observe your body and how you breathe. Do you notice your chest or stomach moving? Many men breathe mostly with their chest, although using your diaphragm ("stomach") is more natural, allowing deeper and more relaxed breathing. Imagine your belly is a balloon, filling up and letting out the air. Exaggerate it. With practice, deep breathing enhances your relaxation.

INDIVIDUAL EXERCISE: Physical Relaxation

Make yourself very comfortable in a chair, sofa, or bed, loosening any tight clothing. Close your eyes and relax. Breathe deeply and slowly, gradually inhaling as you slowly count to five, then exhaling to the count of five.

Relax your toes and feet. Now let the tension in your calves disappear. Imagine a soothing feeling rising through your legs, through your knees to your thighs. Let your legs feel completely relaxed and free of tension. Breathe calmly, deeply, and feel the air move slowly in and out of your body.

Now focus on your pelvis. Let your muscles relax; let go of tension. Let this soothing feeling move through your buttocks. Feel yourself breathing deeply as the tension in the lower half of your body disappears. Then let the tension in your back begin to disappear. Let this soothing feeling wrap around your chest, shoulders, neck, down your arms and hands. Let the relaxation move through your face, feeling your facial muscles relax as you breathe calmly. Feel the tension disappear from your forehead, eyebrows, jaws. Allow your body and mind to feel relaxed and comfortable.

Although this is an individual exercise, you and your partner can do it side by side. Rebecca and Troy found it helpful to make a recording (about five minutes long) of the relaxation instructions. By listening to the recording, they could concentrate more easily. They did the relaxation exercise five times. This was good enough, and they were ready to move to step three.

Step Three: Relaxing Your Pelvic Muscle (PM)

Goal: Identify and learn to consciously use your pelvic muscle for physical relaxation.

This is the "don't be a tightass if you want to relax well enough for easy erections" skill. Your body tightens in response to the pressures, tensions, and burdens of life. This includes unconsciously tightening your *pelvic muscle* (PM). By learning to relax it, you give your body the foundation for easy erections. If your PM relaxes, the rest of your body will follow.

The easiest way to locate your PM is to imagine you are squeezing off urination or "twitching" your penis. You'll feel a mild sensation in one or more of the following areas: your penis, groin, the perineal area (between your testicles and anus), the gluteus maximus (butt) muscles, or the anus.

INDIVIDUAL EXERCISE: PM Basic Training

This exercise will improve your conscious awareness of the sensations of your PM and strengthen the muscle. Contract (tighten) your PM and hold for three seconds, then relax it for three seconds while you consciously focus on the sensations. Do this ten times—tightening three seconds, relaxing three seconds.

Do this set (contracting and relaxing your PM ten times) at three different times every day. At first it may be difficult to tighten and hold the muscle for three seconds, but do what you can (one or two seconds) and build up your strength over time.

INDIVIDUAL EXERCISE: The PM Continuum

This exercise will increase awareness of the sensation of your PM and increase your mental control of your PM. Visualize that your PM can be tightened in varying degrees of intensity. Imagine a continuum from 0 to 10, at first with three stops: 0 (relaxed), 5 (medium), and 10 (tight). Practice moving from one point to another, holding the PM at that level for three seconds, then relax. For example, tighten the PM to 10 and hold for three seconds, then return to 0 for three seconds, then tighten to 5 and hold for three seconds, and then relax to 0. Practice this until it becomes easy. Once you learn this, extend the continuum from three stopping points to five stopping points (10—0—5—0—7—0—3—0). This will be good enough.

Troy was taught to monitor his level of overall relaxation during sex by ensuring his PM was between 1 and 3. Dr. Sawyer told Troy that if his PM was tighter than 3, he was not relaxed enough to expect an easy erection. Dr. Sawyer also instructed Rebecca to relax her PM. She could use graduated tightening of her PM during arousal to help pleasure Troy's penis during intercourse as well as help herself to reach orgasm more easily.

PHASE TWO: ENHANCING YOUR AROUSAL AND EROTIC FLOW

In this phase, you will learn how to increase your pleasure with touch and provide sufficient physiological relaxation and physical stimulation for erections. Using self-entrancement arousal, you will have easy erections, an alternative to the typically impatient and zealous erections of partner interaction arousal. You'll regain confidence, enjoy working cooperatively with your partner, and learn how to build an erotic flow that is strong yet flexible.

Step Four: Relaxed Couple Pleasuring

Goal: Enjoy relaxed, nonerotic, sensual touch.

We literally *need* physical touch. Studies indicate that healthy touch reduces anxiety (Olson and Sneed 1995), soothes and eases grief (Robinson 1996), and reduces frustration (Diego et al. 2002). In a healthy, intimate relationship, touch and sexuality are well integrated. Expanding your awareness and increasing the variety and balance of the types of touch that you give and receive will enrich your sensual and sexual pleasure.

COUPLE EXERCISE: Touch Quality

Discuss the five types of touch below. Then estimate the percent that each type contributes to total touch in your relationship. Then rate the percent of each touch type you want to share in the future. Appreciate your different perspectives, and discuss how you can blend your desires. Discuss how you'd like to alternate the amounts of each touch from time to time, from mood to mood. This helps you create different sensual and sexual scenarios.

Touch Type	Current Percent of Touch		Percent of Touch You Want	
	He	She	He	She
Affectionate Touch: clothes on; warm, friendly, gentle touch; hugging; kissing; holding hands				
Sensual Touch: cuddling, pleasant, cozy, relaxing, soothing; embracing; nongenital touching				
Playful Touch: comfortable, secure—mixing nongenital and genital touching				
Erotic Touch: manual, oral, rubbing —erotic stimulation to orgasm				

Intercourse Touch: penis-vagina connection and bond				

COUPLE EXERCISE: Relaxed Pleasuring

The goal of this exercise is to explore the sensations in your bodies, increase pleasure, and overcome the barriers impeding the relaxed flow of healthy sexual response. This exercise invites you to enjoy *sensual* touch and shows that touch can be pleasurable without being sexually arousing.

Set aside one hour and choose a private, softly lit, warm, and comfortable place. Undress and prepare yourself to be relaxed and focused. For fifteen minutes, pleasure the entire back of your partner's nude body; then, for fifteen minutes, pleasure the front of her body with the exception of her breasts and genitals. Then have her reciprocate, spending fifteen minutes on your back, then fifteen minutes on your front, again avoiding the area around your nipples and genitals. This touch is not intended as massage (designed to loosen up tight muscles) but a relaxed, comforting, sensual touch—a pleasuring.

Keep your attention on your body, focusing upon the sensations you feel as you are being touched or are touching. Feel free to guide your partner by giving verbal appreciation ("Your touching makes me feel warm and secure," "I really like what you are doing now," "Your kisses on my shoulder are so soothing") or taking her hand and nonverbally directing how you want to be touched. If your partner caresses you in a manner that does not please you, take responsibility to speak up. Instead of complaining, you might say, "It feels better when you touch more gently," or "I would enjoy a slow, soft touch now." Otherwise, let the time be quiet, so that you can concentrate on the sensations and pleasurable feelings. If your body responds with an erection, you probably are overdoing the touch, touching too close to erotic areas, or allowing partner interaction arousal ("little erotic movies"). If you are relaxing with the pleasure, you will not feel sexually aroused or erect. If you do become aroused, simply focus on the pleasurable sensations, and your excitement will subside.

Touch for yourself and feel free to experiment with sensations. Touch, hold, kiss, lick, suck, or otherwise caress your partner's body. You may want to explore the joy of touch by using massage oil or talcum powder, or by caressing with feathers, silk, fleece, or flannel.

While you are receiving, selfishly soak up every sensation. Enjoy your here-and-now experience. Concentrate on your own feelings, whether you're giving or receiving. Although pleasing your partner is an important part of a sensual encounter, pleasing yourself is equally important.

Do not use this exercise as an introduction to sex. Not having sex for at least three hours afterward will help protect the relaxing nature of this exercise. If your mind and body anticipate sex, this will become a distraction. Remember, this is a sensual relaxation exercise.

When you and your partner are able to comfortably relax, focus on the sensual pleasure, limit mental distractions to less than 20 percent of the time, and not experience erotic response (erection), you are ready to move on to the next step.

Troy and Rebecca did four sessions of this relaxed pleasuring exercise. At first, to Troy's surprise, he would get an erection by simply pleasuring Rebecca's legs, thighs, or stomach. Troy changed focus to what he was feeling in his fingers (sensual self-entrancement arousal) as he touched her and avoided looking at Rebecca's breasts or genitals and fantasizing (partner interaction arousal).

Step Five: Your Cognitive Map for Erotic Flow

Goal: Develop awareness of the range of your sexual arousal.

This exercise provides the grounding for guiding your erotic flow. By developing a cognitive map, you'll understand how to develop your erotic flow, blend self-entrancement arousal and partner interaction arousal, and ensure you will maintain an erection during lovemaking.

Each of us has our own sexual arousal patterns or desired sequences that blend reality and imagination. By understanding the erotic flow evoked by specific images, behaviors, and feelings, you can consciously modify eroticism in order to slow down, hold steady, or intensify your arousal. This is a tool that can help you blend the arousal styles.

INDIVIDUAL EXERCISE: Developing Your Erotic Continuum

Create your map of arousal by making a detailed, specific list of images, feelings, behaviors, techniques, and scenarios that you find arousing. Using a scale of 1 to 100, with 100 equaling ejaculation (orgasm), assign an arousal level to each. Be sure to develop the 1-to-50 range of items instead of jumping to the higher items. On his list of twenty-five specific items, Troy assigned closed-lip kissing 15, fondling Rebecca's breasts with clothes on 35, Rebecca gently stroking his penis 60, and fondling her naked breasts while Rebecca gently stroked his penis 75.

When you experience ED, one of several problems involving erotic flow usually occurs. It may be that your erotic flow is obstructed or derailed by distractions, fatigue, performance anxiety, or spectatoring. You may be outpacing your erotic flow by engaging in sex too frantically or passionately. We call this sexual drag racing. This occurs when you begin sex at a point of 50 or more and rush arousal. This "champing at the bit" can create ED through performance anxiety. Remember the guideline for functional erections: Integrate your level of physical relaxation with a *graduated* level of physical and cognitive stimulation.

Step Six: Partner Genital Exploration and Comfort

Goal: Learn more about your own sensations and your partner's; enjoy calm, relaxed touch and physical relaxation in an otherwise erotic situation.

This exercise sets the foundation for building your couple erotic flow. You will take turns leading each other in an exploration of your genitals. The purpose is to provide a sensual exploration of your body's erotic parts, to practice sexual leadership with your own body, and to become more comfortable looking at and touching each other's genitals in a relaxing, nonarousing way. This exercise is a show-and-tell about your body and erogenous zones. Remember that this is fundamentally a relaxation exercise.

COUPLE EXERCISE: Partner Genital Exploration

This exercise will take approximately one hour. Begin with thirty minutes (fifteen minutes for each of you) of relaxed nongenital pleasuring (this is a shortened version of the relaxed couple pleasuring exercise you learned in step four).

Have your partner lie comfortably in a reclining position, propped up on her back with pillows. Position yourself comfortably alongside her, facing her. For the next fifteen minutes, have her lead you in an exploration of her erogenous parts.

Do not pursue arousal. Discuss the sensations, what she prefers for relaxation, and what is uncomfortable. Discuss how you can enrich her pleasure. Ask questions of each other to learn or confirm what you experience. Use a scale of 1 to 10 to talk about how erotically sensitive a particular area is.

Gently explore the sensations of her breasts, nipples, stomach, hips, upper thighs, inner thighs, outer lips of her vagina, perineum (the area between her vagina and anus), clitoris, and inside her vagina. Many women have uncomfortable feelings about this, associating it with a gynecological exam, so let her take the lead. Be sure she feels comfortable and in control. Give her your hand and ask her to direct your touch. She might have you form a Y-shape with your index and middle finger and show you how to gently pleasure the outer lips of her vagina. Talk, describe, and discuss.

When you are ready to explore sensations inside her vagina, have her guide you in inserting one of your fingers and direct you. Imagine her vagina as the face of a clock, with the top being 12:00. Have her slowly guide your pleasuring. Many women find they feel very little beyond three-quarters to one inch inside. Proceed around the face of the clock to 3:00, 6:00, and 9:00, stopping at each point, exploring and discussing the sensations. Work cooperatively to learn, confirm, relax, and enjoy.

Now it is your turn. Take the lead in the exploration of your body. Begin with your chest and nipples. Take your partner's hand and direct her, using the 1-to-10 scale to note the level of sensitivity you feel. Be sure you feel comfortable, especially when she is exploring your testicles. You might have her cup one or both testicles and describe for her your sensations, or ask her to explore different parts with her finger, showing her how to pleasure you. Women have heard that men's testicles are very delicate. Be sure to teach her about your testicles so she is not over- or undersensitive. Then have her gently place your penis back onto your stomach. Ask her to take her index finger and, beginning at the base of your penis, very slowly explore sensations up the penile shaft. Show her the sensitive parts on your penis, sharing what you are feeling.

Do this exercise a minimum of three times before moving to the next step. The repetition will increase your comfort and allow you to feel calm.

Rebecca and Troy engaged in the "Partner Genital Exploration" exercise four times. Both were surprised that a calm sensual feeling in their genitals developed while in a relaxed state. This was quite a change from what they expected and from what occurred the first time they tried the exercise. At first, Troy found it difficult to not get an erotic movie going in his imagination (partner interaction arousal), and this, he observed later, caused an erection. It increased his awareness of the power of partner interaction arousal.

COUPLE EXERCISE: Playful Nicknames for Your Special Sexual Parts

Many couples have private nicknames for each other's sexual parts. For example, his penis may be "Big Ben" (the clock tower in London), "the Monument" (referring to the Washington Monument), or "Lollipop." Or her breasts may be the "Grand Tetons" (mountain peaks in Wyoming) and her genitals "my penis warmer" or "Powder Puff." The important thing is that the nickname be tender and affirming. Sarcasm is not playful unless you are teasing yourself. For example, a man having difficulty gaining an erection might ask her if she'd "kiss my miniature penis for a while to see if he'll salute." Be playful, but remember the bedroom is the most sensitive place in our lives.

Do you have special, playful, private names for your own and your partner's sexual parts? What makes a nickname comfortable and endearing? What nicknames would you like to create or prefer to use?

Step Seven: Couple Arousal Training: Easy Erections

Goal: Learn to enjoy your easy erection, then choose to let it go, then comfortably regain it.

This exercise will show you how easy it is to get an erection, let it subside, and regain it when you stay relaxed and focus on self-entrancement arousal. You are balancing the two physical conditions your body needs for erection: relaxation and stimulation. You'll want to practice this exercise several times, until you again feel confident with your erections.

COUPLE EXERCISE: Wax and Wane

This exercise has three stages, and you'll want to practice each stage more than once. Begin each session by doing relaxed couple pleasuring for thirty minutes.

1. Soothing Genital Touch
   Rest on your back and ask your partner to gently and soothingly explore your testicles and penis with soft, slow touch for fifteen minutes. Concentrate on the quiet, calm sensations. Relax your PM. She can give you featherlike touching or fingering to pleasure your penis but *without producing an erection*. Relax and concentrate on the calm sensations. Do this exercise at least twice.

2. Finding Your Calm, Easy Erection
After thirty minutes of relaxed couple pleasuring, have your partner gently touch your genitals in a relaxing way. Then ask her to very gradually increase her fingering of your penis. Do not work to obtain an erection, but very slowly *allow* an erection by continuing your relaxation, keeping your PM relaxed, and focusing on the pleasure in your penis. The more relaxed and focused you are, the easier it will become erect. You are practicing getting an erection with self-entrancement arousal—maximum body relaxation, minimal touch, and focus on your sensations (without partner interaction focus or fantasy).

Be patient. Typically, it will take at least five to ten minutes before an erection begins. Do not press it, or you will become distracted by spectatoring and undermine your physical relaxation. After several minutes of calm touch, she can increase the stimulation just a little. You are waiting to find the *minimum* touch you require to get an erection. Be sure you are not rushing it, because you would conclude that you need more stimulation than is really necessary. Keep your PM relaxed and let her gradually increase penile touch. She may add stimulation by gently using both hands.

If after three exercises you have not begun to find your calm erection, then you may begin to add mildly arousing partner interaction fantasy. Look at your partner, or choose an item in the less arousing range of your continuum. You are searching for the *mildest* physical (self-entrancement) and cognitive (partner involvement) arousals that you need for an easy erection. When your calm erection begins, enjoy it.

3. Choosing to Wax and Wane
This time, repeat stage two, and after you've had an erection for three to five minutes, choose to let it subside about 50 percent by stopping or changing the penile touch. As you feel your erection subsiding, stay focused on your sensations. Then signal her to change the touch to gradually bring back a relaxed erection. Notice that when you're physically relaxed, it is easier to regain your erection. You can lose your erection and regain it easily when you are calm and focused.

Troy worked too hard during this exercise, until he realized he was trying to rush an erection rather than waiting for it to occur. Dr. Sawyer reminded him to maintain a relaxed PM. Rebecca invited him to be patient and let her provide the pleasure. It was difficult for Troy to be completely passive; he felt he didn't deserve the exclusive attention. Eventually, the exercise went well, and Troy gained comfort with easy erections.

What If You Have Trouble with Easy Erections?

If you find that an easy erection does not occur during the "Wax and Wane" exercise, then practice this exercise on your own. After you have successfully done this, you can repeat the exercise with your partner.

PHASE THREE: ENJOYING CONFIDENT AND FLEXIBLE INTERCOURSE

Now that you've expanded your comfort with your body and your partner and learned relaxation and self-entrancement arousal, you're ready to expand your pleasure by learning to have intercourse with confidence and flexibility.

Step Eight: Progressive Intercourse

Goal: Integrate the skills and become confident with erections during intercourse.

This exercise reinforces the idea that pleasuring, eroticism, arousal, and intercourse are parts of a continuous, flowing process. We invite you to think of intercourse as a special pleasuring experience within this process.

COUPLE EXERCISE: Initiating Intercourse

Begin by doing relaxed couple pleasuring for thirty minutes. Then lie on your back and invite your partner to straddle you and gently pleasure your penis to bring about an easy erection. When you have an erection and when she wishes, she can take your penis and insert you into her vagina.

You do nothing but relax and focus on the pleasure. She can comfortably move up and down to maintain your erection. Do not proceed to orgasm. Enjoy this close and pleasurable intercourse for ten to fifteen minutes, then gradually slow and stop, and enjoy cuddling as a way to end the session. Complete this exercise a minimum of two times. In subsequent exercises, allow intercourse to promote an erotic flow which naturally culminates in orgasm (ejaculation).

What If You Have Trouble with Initiating Intercourse?

The most common point at which men have trouble with the graduated steps is at the moment of initiating intercourse. This is expected, because that is the point at which performance anxiety peaks, especially when you still adhere to the detrimental belief that sex equals intercourse and view intercourse as the moment of truth. Challenge this self-defeating belief and remind yourself that you now know how to get and keep an erection. Relaxing your body and focusing on pleasure is key. Allow your partner to lead; you just sit back and let her manage initiating intercourse. Remember that she is your intimate sexual friend who wants you to experience pleasure and satisfaction.

If your difficulty continues, another option to consider is using a proerection medication (Cialis, Levitra, or Viagra) to help overcome performance anxiety. When you are comfortable with intercourse, you can gradually phase out the medication.

When you complete the "Initiating Intercourse" exercise three times with good-enough erections, then you can learn the "stuff-it" method as an additional enjoyable technique. We offer you this method so you can enjoy intercourse free of performance anxiety.

COUPLE EXERCISE: The "Stuff-It" Method

Begin with thirty minutes of relaxed pleasuring, and then lie on your back as your partner straddles you. It may help if you place a pillow under your hips to raise up for her. If you get an erection, wait until it goes down so you can begin intercourse without an erection. Focusing only on your sensations and keeping your PM relaxed, allow your partner to insert ("stuff") your flaccid penis into the lips of her vagina. This may seem strange at first, but if she adjusts her position as she straddles you while gently sitting down on your genital area, she can take your flaccid penis between her thumb and fingers, and using her other hand to hold open the lips of her vagina, maneuver her hips so she can insert you. This will require cooperation—maneuvering, scrunching, and angling.

Once inside, remain still and let her sit on you and gently pleasure your penis inside the lips of her vagina. Enjoy the contact as she moves ever so slowly and with downward pressure. Pay attention to the subtle pleasure, because if she moves too much, you'll plop out. If this happens, let her simply reinsert your penis. Have intercourse this way for ten minutes. If you are sufficiently relaxed (remember to monitor your PM), you will eventually start to gain an erection. Allow it to occur and enjoy the special closeness, but do not go on to orgasm.

If after two exercises you have not gained an erection inside her vagina, allow yourself to include sufficient partner interaction arousal by choosing an item from your erotic flow map such as watching your partner on top of you or touching her.

How does it feel to begin intercourse this way? Strange? Warm? Embarrassing? Intimate? How does it feel for you to have your erection growing inside her vagina? For her? When might you want to begin intercourse this way?

Troy and Rebecca found initiating intercourse anxiety provoking because they worried about performance pressure. Yet Troy did fine, and this confirmed for him the need for physical relaxation and graduated stimulation. He was especially relieved to learn the stuff-it method, and he felt reassured that Rebecca really liked it, saying how close and cuddly she felt.

Step Nine: Intimate and Flexible Intercourse

Goal: Enjoy intercourse, encourage your partner's pleasure, and develop alternative (nonintercourse) scenarios.

COUPLE EXERCISE: Enjoying Intercourse

Begin with relaxed couple pleasuring, and have your partner help you obtain an erection. Then share mutual pleasuring, including manual and oral stimulation, blending sensual self-entrancement with partner interaction focus. Allow the pleasuring to be slow, tender, caring, and rhythmic. Then lie comfortably on your back on the bed, with your partner straddling you.

Let the transition to intercourse be unhurried and flowing, allowing her to guide intromission. Then she can begin the type of thrusting she finds most arousing—slow up-and-down, circular, or rhythmic in-and-out. You can utilize your greater freedom to caress, stroke, fondle, and kiss her body throughout intercourse. Multiple stimulation during intercourse can facilitate arousal for both of you. This can include gentle clitoral stimulation, whether by your hands, her hands, or indirect stimulation from coital movement. Be aware of what is most arousing for you and stay with the erotic flow. Experiment, cooperate, and give feedback to find ways to establish mutually enjoyable intercourse. Enjoy the entire pleasuring, arousal, and intercourse process for about an hour, and complete the exercise at least twice.

Experiment with variations of man-on-top intercourse. We suggest spending more time than usual on pleasuring; allow arousal to be at least 7 or 8 on a scale of 1 to 10 before transitioning to intercourse. Avoid switching to intercourse as soon as you're erect. If you've enjoyed multiple stimulation during the pleasuring and eroticism phase, then continue this during intercourse. Enjoy a building eroticism throughout intercourse. You can kiss, you can fondle her breasts, she can stimulate your testicles or buttocks, and you can scratch her back or stroke her thighs.

Throughout, take care to balance sensual self-entrancement arousal with partner interaction arousal in order to sustain your erection and not ejaculate before you want to. Balancing arousal styles is especially important if your ED was accompanied by premature ejaculation. Feel free to utilize fantasies (cognitive partner interaction arousal) to enhance arousal and erotic flow. Experiment with position variations: having her legs fully elevated and resting on your shoulders, putting a pillow under her buttocks to adjust the vaginal angle, having her lock her legs around your body.

Developing Flexible Scenarios

Enjoying flexible couple sexuality includes intimate intercourse as well as erotic, nonintercourse backup scenarios and sensual, close backup scenarios. Good-enough sex involves pleasuring which flows to intercourse most but not all of the time.

You can learn to accept that not every sexual experience needs to end in intercourse. Variability will enhance your sexual desire, not inhibit it. Manual, oral, rubbing, and penile stimulation are excellent ways to experience high arousal and orgasm for one or both of you. In truth, the majority of women find it easier to be orgasmic with manual and oral stimulation. Orgasm reached through erotic, nonintercourse stimulation can be satisfying for your partner and for you.

A key to intimate sexuality is awareness that there are a number of ways to give and receive pleasure. It's not necessary to feel anxious, panic, and try to force your penis into her vagina. Don't give in to performance anxiety. Stay actively involved in the sexual give-and-take. You can request oral stimulation to enhance erotic flow, or focus on stimulating her so you can piggyback your arousal on hers. Feel free to pause intercourse and relax or talk together. Then you can slowly increase arousal, rebuild your erotic flow, and return to intercourse. Remember what you learned in the "Wax and Wane" exercise: There is more than one erection in you if you stay relaxed. Don't panic, fearing your erection is lost forever. Relax, refocus with gentle touch, and your erection will easily return.

Sometimes, an encounter will not involve erotic response or intercourse. Rather than feeling frustrated or withdrawing, either of you can say that this will not be a sexual night, and you can end the encounter with affectionate and sensual touching and intimacy. When this happens, make a commitment to have a sexual encounter in the next one to three days when you have the time and energy for a relaxed erotic experience.

COUPLE EXERCISE: Developing Flexible Scenarios

Take a moment to think about three sexual scenarios you would enjoy. Prod yourself to be creative and flexible by allowing only one of the three to include intercourse. Then take turns sharing these scenarios, alternating one at a time. Be careful not to judge but to enjoy.

Step 10: Sexual Playfulness

Goal: Create fun and enjoyment with sex.

Sexually satisfied couples value a certain amount of adult playfulness, whether humor, lightheartedness, affectionate teasing, sexual nicknames, or intellectual bantering. Mature playfulness also has a deeper intimacy-building side, including sharing memories of unique times, traditions, special moments, private meanings, even spirituality. The way you play together makes you unique and special as a couple.

Sex is a form of healthy, adult playfulness. For sex to be playful, it must be kind and caring, respectful and accepting, and safe and secure. Teasing yourself is fine, but teasing your partner is risky.

Intimacy deepens when you know your partner well enough to understand in what ways she is comfortable experimenting with your bodies and sexual scenarios. On an intimate level, playfulness signals that the feelings of closeness are more important than anything else (for example, performance) and that your relationship is special. Play brings us full circle to our primary goal: relationship intimacy.

COUPLE EXERCISE: Alternative Scenarios

Expand your comfort with an innovative sexual scenario. This exercise will help you decide on an activity you want to cultivate and ensure a sense of trust within your erotic scenario. This means talking with your partner about what you will do and deciding on a signal to pause or stop should it stretch your comfort level too far. Approach this activity gradually. With repetition, you will find that your emotional comfort and pleasure will grow.

Choose scenarios from the following list that you may occasionally want to incorporate into your lovemaking, or create your own. There are no right or wrong desires, only individual preferences. Talk about these scenarios. Do not present your desire as a demand. Remember that everyone has areas of shyness and discomfort. You have a right to say no to a sexual scenario. Using a scale of 1 to 10, rate your respective levels of interest and then your levels of comfort. Evaluate your comfort by the three criteria for intimate play: caring, respect, and security. Then decide what you'll try. Use this exercise as an opportunity to think boldly of yourself as a sexual person who has the right to pleasure and joy.

Playful Scenario	Level of Interest		Level of Comfort	
	He	She	He	She
Playing strong or aggressive, shy or hard-to-get				
Wearing sexy lingerie or briefs				
Talking "dirty" during sex				
Playful bondage (for example, hands tied with crepe paper)				
Sex in special places (before the fireplace, car, beach)				
Holding hands while you have intercourse				
Acting naughty or wild				
Using "toys" like oils, dildo, feathers, or vibrator				
Pretend that you are virgins having sex for the first time				
Take turns performing a striptease for each other				
Have phone sex				
Take turns with "her night" and "his night" when you can request a special erotic scenario				

Watch an X-rated DVD/video as the entrée to your lovemaking				
Gaze into each other's eyes during intercourse				

Troy and Rebecca discussed a number of items and discovered that they both were interested in wearing sexy lingerie and briefs—Troy rating an interest of 7, Rebecca a 6. Troy also wished Rebecca to dance for him wearing the lingerie, which she was less interested in, feeling shy. Rebecca wanted Troy to wear silk briefs and hold his crotch and invite her to explore what was there. They agreed to try this and decided that during the first exploration, Rebecca would dance suggestively for thirty seconds, then Troy would stand before her and invite her to explore his crotch for thirty seconds. If either were to say, "I want to stop for now," they would immediately stop and hug, no questions asked, and later share how they felt.

Rebecca said she enjoyed being seductive, feeling proud that Troy seemed very pleased. Troy revealed that he felt embarrassed. They agreed to repeat the exploration in a week, Rebecca wanting to dance for a full minute and Troy wanting to keep his crotch exploration invitation to the same thirty seconds. With repetition, each increased comfort and expressed feelings of sexual self-esteem and enjoyed their couple eroticism. They decided to incorporate this new scenario into their lovemaking several times a year at either's request.

WHAT IF THESE SKILLS DON'T WORK FOR YOU?

While this program is helpful for most men and couples, do not be discouraged if some of the exercises do not work as well for you. If you get stuck, it would be wise to consult an experienced sex therapist to help you develop your own way to integrate the skills for increasing confidence with erections and ensuring sexual growth and satisfaction.

9

Developing Your Couple Sexual Style

Now that you have worked as an intimate team to build comfort and confidence with erections, it is time to consider how sexuality fits into the "big picture" of your relationship. You owe it to yourself and your partner to develop a comfortable, pleasurable, and functional couple sexual style. This will help you maintain the progress you've made and will strengthen your long-term sexual and relationship satisfaction. Healthy sexuality is an intimate team effort, not an individual sexual performance. Emotional and sexual intimacy are the glue of your couple bond. Your emotional relationship is the energy source for a vital, satisfying sexuality.

It is important to find a mutually comfortable level of intimacy that promotes sexual desire and initiation. The traditional belief was that the more emotional intimacy, the better the marriage. In fact, that is a myth. A crucial factor in developing a couple style is maintaining a balance between autonomy and intimacy.

In this chapter, we will explore the common marital styles and the role sexuality plays in each. We will examine both strengths and potential problems of each couple style. We will also examine dating and serious relationships and the role of sexuality in these. Finally, we'll guide you through consciously choosing a couple style that works for you.

MARITAL AND SEXUAL STYLES

There are four marital styles, each of which takes a specific approach to intimacy, autonomy, communication, power dynamics, and conflict resolution. In their order of frequency, they are *complementary, conflict-minimizing, best friend,* and *emotionally expressive.* Of course, these are not pure categories, but one style does predominate for each couple.

The Complementary Couple Style

The complementary couple style is the most common. Each partner respects the other's contributions, each has his or her domain of competence and power, and each values moderate intimacy balanced by a clear sense of autonomy. These couples are able to resolve conflicts and maintain dialogue about difficult issues. Each partner feels valued, respected, and cared for. The emotional tone of the relationship is affirming.

Complementary couples have a good sexual relationship, seeing sexuality as a positive, integral component of their marital bond but certainly not the most important factor. The trap for this marital style is to fall into a pattern of routine, mechanical sex. Sex becomes a low priority, occurring late at night after all the "important" things in life are done (like putting the children to sleep, paying bills, walking the dog). Sex might be functional (for instance, the man maintains a good erection), but it lacks excitement and emotional intimacy. The couple thinks about their early sexual experiences—and possibly their experiences working together to overcome ED—and they miss that sense of connection and specialness. Another danger, especially with the aging of the people and the marriage, is that their focus on intercourse subverts satisfaction.

Ideally, each spouse would be comfortable initiating and each would feel free to decline and perhaps offer an alternative way to connect. Maintaining a vital sexual relationship is a couple task, with the woman's sexual feelings and "voice" playing an integral role.

The Conflict-Minimizing Couple Style

The conflict-minimizing couple style is the most stable. These marriages are typically organized along traditional gender roles, with the man as the prime income generator and the woman the homemaker, although other patterns are common in recent years. These marriages are characterized by avoidance of strong emotional expression (especially anger), limited intimacy, and emphasis on children, family, and religious values. The emotional and practical rules of the marriage are clearly understood and consistently implemented. Conflict-minimizing couples value security over intimacy and family over coupleness. People value this marital style because of its predictability and security.

The role of sex is de-emphasized. The limited emotional expression can result in inhibited erotic expression. Sexual problems are typically minimized.

Initiating sex and establishing sexual frequency is the man's role. The sexual scenario emphasizes intercourse, with one-way foreplay rather than mutual pleasuring. The expectation is that she will function like him: have a single orgasm during intercourse with no additional stimulation. Sex is his domain; affection is her domain.

There are several possible sexual traps within this marital style. The biggest is that sex becomes marginal and mechanical, and eventually infrequent. The couple falls into the cycle of a low-sex or no-sex marriage. Another trap is that the sole focus on intercourse makes the man vulnerable to ED. The couple have not been intimate friends, which makes it hard to develop intimate, interactive sexuality.

Conflict-minimizing couples miss the opportunity to use differences and conflicts to deepen intimacy, and they underestimate the role of sexuality in energizing their marital bond. We urge couples who choose this marital style to be sure that sexuality, including enjoying erections and intercourse, plays a 15 to 20 percent role in marital vitality and satisfaction.

The Best Friend Couple Style

The best friend style is characterized by the highest degree of intimacy, acceptance, and sharing; equitable distribution of roles and responsibilities; and a commitment to a close, vital marriage. Although the cultural ideal, this marital style runs the risk of leading to disappointment and alienation when emotional and sexual expectations are not met or there are irresolvable conflicts.

When both individuals choose this marital style and devote the time and psychological energy to make it successful, this is a very impressive marriage. However, best friend couples have a high divorce rate, based on disappointment and resentment toward the spouse and the marriage.

For a best friend couple, sex energizes the relationship and makes it special. They enjoy touching both inside and outside the bedroom. Intimacy, pleasuring, and eroticism are valued by both people. Their sexual style is flexible and responsive to the feelings and preferences of both partners.

The biggest emotional trap is enmeshment, meaning that they sacrifice autonomy and individuality for the sake of the relationship. When things do not work well, they regress to hurt, blaming, and resentment. Disappointment and disillusion rob the marriage of vitality. These couples usually lack conflict resolution skills and become bitter over thwarted hopes and expectations.

The biggest sexual trap is inhibited sexual desire. Intimacy and couple time serve as bridges to sexual desire, but too much intimacy can stifle erotic feelings. Best friend couples are not assertive in dealing with sexual problems. They expect each should know what the other is thinking and what the other wants without having to ask or articulate. When there is a sexual dysfunction, especially ED, love and communication are not enough. Warm feelings and caring communication are helpful, but you need more to overcome ED and rebuild satisfying couple sexuality. The combination of taking personal responsibility and working as an intimate sexual team can be a challenge for best friend couples.

The Emotionally Expressive Couple Style

The emotionally expressive couple style is the most volatile and unstable but also the most engaging, fun, and erotic. Intimacy is like an accordion: sometimes very close, other times very distant. Emotionally expressive couples have the highest intensity of feelings, both loving and angry. They value intimacy and vitality without being afraid of conflict or anger. When this style works well, it can be the framework for a vibrant and exciting relationship. Emotionally expressive couples value sexuality that is spontaneous, adventuresome, playful, and energizing.

Unfortunately, this is the most unstable marital style, the most likely to result in divorce. The conflicts are frequent and intense. Emotionally expressive couples can deal with disappointment, anger, and conflict, but if they cross the line into personal put-downs, contempt, and disrespect, this breaks the bond.

There are a number of potential sexual problems, including using sex to make up after an abusive fight. It is poisonous for physical and emotional fights to serve as foreplay for sex. Another problem is that a gradual, step-by-step approach to dealing with ED—or a relapse—is difficult because they want a spontaneous, freewheeling approach. If the sexual problem can't be resolved quickly, they become demoralized, bitter, and blaming.

To avoid these traps, the emotionally expressive couple needs to respect personal and sexual boundaries. If ED or another sexual dysfunction develops, the couple must address it cooperatively and without rancor.

CHOOSING A MARITAL AND SEXUAL STYLE

It is important to choose a couple style that reflects the way you'd like to deal with intimacy and conflicts, and to adopt a sexual style that is compatible with—and hopefully enhances—your marital style. Mutual endorsement of your chosen couple style is very important. It is not the man's (or woman's) decision to make alone, but a cooperative choice based on respect and empathy for each person's preferences and values.

The two most important issues to address are the amount of emotional intimacy and the importance of sexuality. Emotional intimacy is the degree and quality of personal self-disclosure and empathy. Sexual intimacy includes affectionate, sensual, playful, and erotic touch in addition to intercourse. An example of a problematic intimacy and sexuality pattern is when one spouse (typically the woman) desires high levels of emotional intimacy, while the other spouse wants sex to be the main source of connection. These couples fall into the distancer-versus-pursuer trap, and both forms of intimacy suffer. You can choose instead to cooperate to enhance emotional and sexual intimacy.

EXERCISE: Choosing Your Relationship Style

Consider the following questions individually, then share your thoughts and work together to choose a mutually acceptable couple style. To make this more concrete, write your responses down.

How much emotional intimacy do you want in your life and relationship?

What are the most important emotions you want to share in your relationship?

What is your preferred way to deal with differences and conflicts?

What is your preferred couple style: complementary, conflict-minimizing, best friend, emotionally expressive?

What are the strengths and vulnerabilities of the style you chose?

■ Joshua and Melinda

Forty-six-year-old Joshua made a private deal with himself: If he could overcome ED, he would do anything Melinda wanted. Joshua had struggled with ED for six years, and it had grown more severe and more draining of his self-esteem and the closeness in their relationship. He had tried the usual unsuccessful coping strategies: minimize the problem, blame Melinda's heavier body, use a potency enhancer from a natural food store, get a Viagra prescription from his internist, surf the Internet for porn sites to boost his desire. Finally, Joshua felt ready to share with Melinda his sense of sexual despair. Paradoxically, Melinda felt relieved. She had worried that Joshua was having an affair. The fact that Joshua was offended by this shows how emotionally disconnected and misunderstood each person felt.

Luckily, Joshua and Melinda realized right away that they would need to treat ED as their common enemy. Melinda accompanied Joshua to an appointment with the internist, Dr. Bennis, who was surprised to hear that Viagra had not helped. She assumed that his erections were fine since Joshua had not mentioned the problem again. She scheduled a full physical for Joshua and invited Melinda to the follow-up meeting.

Dr. Bennis found no major physical problem, but she did strongly recommend a number of health changes. She suggested that Joshua go on a diet to lose fifteen pounds. She advised him to reduce alcohol consumption from twenty to ten drinks a week, substitute red wine for beer, and have only one or two drinks in the six hours before being sexual. She recommended that Joshua get at least seven hours of sleep every night instead of going to sleep at 1:00 A.M. on weekdays and sleeping ten hours on weekends to catch up. Finally, she recommended that Joshua exercise moderately three to five times a week rather than engaging in hard, competitive exercise for three hours once a week, as had been Joshua's habit. Dr. Bennis's message was that at forty-six, Joshua's body was less forgiving, so he had to adopt better health habits. This would translate to better sexual health. She changed Joshua's prescription to Cialis and gave them a referral to a sex therapist. Melinda agreed to be the "cheerleader" for both the health and sexual change plans.

With the help of the therapist, Joshua and Melinda worked together to change their attitudes and expectations, modify their marital and sexual style, learn new erotic scenarios, and use multiple stimulation during intercourse. They found it helpful to have sex in the morning or afternoon rather than late at night. They found that intercourse worked best when Melinda used a vaginal lubricant and guided intromission.

Joshua and Melinda had been a traditional, conflict-minimizing couple until the advent of ED. An unexpected positive side effect of dealing with ED was that they transitioned to a complementary style. Their sexual relationship now tended more toward the best friend style, although they were careful to ensure that there was enough emotional space for desire and eroticism. Melinda had been frustrated with their old couple style. She had not liked the rigidity of their roles and felt that Joshua had a limited understanding of her strengths and uniqueness. So Melinda was very pleased to have a complementary, equitable marital relationship. Joshua had felt burdened by the traditional role, especially in regard to career and money, but assumed that was simply the reality of being a man. Sharing roles and responsibilities was a relief on one hand, but on the other hand, Joshua was someone who valued tradition and predictability. Joshua found their complementary couple style challenging, although ultimately worthwhile.

The hardest concept for Joshua to accept was the 85 percent good-enough sex guideline. It was a paradox, because he very much enjoyed erotic, nonintercourse sex to orgasm. He especially enjoyed one-way sex. Joshua preferred receiving manual rather than oral stimulation to orgasm. He found this hard to admit to himself, much less to Melinda. She did enjoy being orgasmic with intercourse but also liked manual and oral stimulation to orgasm. She had never felt that orgasm was absolutely necessary for sexual pleasure and satisfaction.

Over time, Joshua and Melinda became more and more satisfied with their new marital and sexual style. Melinda even said she was glad they had to confront ED because in addressing the sexual dysfunction, their marital relationship had become stronger and healthier. Joshua agreed about the marital growth, but he would have preferred to skip the ED problem.

Men in Dating or Living-Together Relationships

Many men with ED are single, divorced, or in cohabitating relationships. How do these couple and sexual styles relate to them? Consider that there are three levels of relationship connection: sexual friendships, lover relationships, and serious relationships. At all levels of a relationship, there are two important guidelines. The first is to treat each other with respect and have an understanding that you will try to not do anything emotionally or sexually that is harmful to her or to yourself. The second is to be realistic about your relationship and not to overpromise or be manipulative.

Sexual friendship is just what it sounds like: You are friends who have a sexual relationship. As with any other friendship, you want to treat the person well, expect to be treated well in turn, and freely share activities and emotions. However, you do not promise a lifelong relationship or change life plans, career, or where you live for the other, nor do you ask this person to make those changes for you. Both people are clear and realistic about their expectations. Whether the relationship lasts six months or three years, the reality is it will end. Hopefully, you wish each other well and remain friends, but there are no guarantees.

The lover relationship involves more closeness, more sharing (you may or may not live together), and more of an emotional investment. Lovers meet each other's families, make long-term vacation and holiday plans, and integrate each other into their lives. However, you do not change your life or career plans for a lover. You do not promise a lifetime commitment or plan to have children in a lover relationship.

The serious relationship has the potential to result in marriage. With time and experience, the relationship grows more intimate and involving. This is the type of relationship in which you consider changing your life in tandem with your partner and discuss all the complicated and sensitive issues involved in sharing your lives emotionally, practically, financially, and sexually.

Issues of respect, trust, and emotional and sexual intimacy are just as relevant for nonmarried as for married couples. Sexuality—including ED—should not make or break the future of the relationship. For example, the fact that the woman helped you regain comfort and confidence with erections does not mean you owe her—or that she owes you—a lifetime commitment. Conversely, struggling with a sexual dysfunction is problematic but need not be a reason to terminate a relationship. As in a marriage, sexuality should play an important but not decisive role.

Developing Your Couple Sexual Style

Establish your unique sexual style by exploring and sharing your sexual desires, feelings, and preferences. This exercise is divided into phases, the first to do individually. Then share your thoughts and work together to reach understandings and agreements.

EXERCISE: Developing Your Couple Sexual Style

Think about and then write out your answers to the following questions. Do not be "politically correct" or try to second-guess your partner. Be honest and explicit.

How important is sex in your life? What role do you want it to play in your relationship?

In terms of affectionate touch, do you prefer kissing, holding hands, or hugging?

How much do you enjoy cuddling? How important is it to you?

How do you distinguish affectionate touch from seductive touch?

How much do you enjoy sensual touch? Do you prefer taking turns or simultaneously giving and receiving?

What is the meaning and value of playful touch? How comfortable are you with affectionate or silly nicknames for your genitals and sexual activities?

How much do you enjoy erotic scenarios and techniques? Do you enjoy erotic sex as a route to orgasm or only as a pleasuring experience?

Do you prefer single stimulation or multiple stimulation? Do you enjoy using external stimuli or not?

What is your preferred intercourse position? Man on top, woman on top, rear entry, side to side? What type of thrusting do you prefer? In and out? Circular? Deep inside? Shallow? Fast or slow?

How much do you value afterplay as a part of your lovemaking style?

Next, read your partner's responses and carefully discuss each question, clarifying both the practical and emotional dimensions. Remember that you are not clones of each other. You want to maintain your individuality and not feel embarrassed or apologetic about your emotional and sexual desires. Your preferences and sensitivities are part of who you are as a sexual person and must be integrated into your couple style for you to be truly satisfied.

Finally, divide your answers into three categories:

Areas you agree on. These will enhance your enjoyment and satisfaction. For example, you both agree that you want sex to play a 15 to 20 percent energizing role, there are no major conflicts, you enjoy sensual and playful touch more than affectionate touch, on occasion you find erotic stimulation to orgasm very exciting, you have three favorite intercourse positions in common, and you value verbally sharing and bonding afterplay.

Areas you can reach agreement on. Identify differences you can accept and even enjoy. Perhaps the spouse who more highly values sex agrees to be the initiator most of the time; one person prefers hugging, the other kissing; one would rather engage in touching standing up and the other prefers sitting down; she likes to talk about feelings and fantasies while he would rather fantasize with his eyes closed and focus on physical sensations; he prefers woman-on-top intercourse while she prefers side-to-side. These are not matters of right and wrong. You can integrate your preferences or take turns. Enjoy your partner's unique sexual preferences. Remember, an involved, aroused partner is the best aphrodisiac.

Differences to accept or adapt to. Finally, there are areas of major differences. For example, one feels sex is the major means of connection and the other emphasizes individual pursuits rather than being a couple; one loves playful touching and the other hates playful touch; she wants to use a vibrator during intercourse to help her be orgasmic, but he is put off by the vibrator; she prefers woman-on-top intercourse, while he prefers rear entry; he likes being sexual late at night in bed, while she likes being sexual in different places in the middle of the day; he wants to experiment with porn videos, which she sees as degrading to women. It is not easy, or even possible, to integrate these differences, but there are two major coping strategies. One is to acknowledge the differences but not let them turn into a power struggle. Instead, accept these and try to work around them. It helps to recognize that difference does not mean rejection. The second strategy is to agree to enter couple therapy to understand the meaning of the differences and find a common ground for intimacy and sexuality.

To develop your comfortable, pleasurable, functional, and mutually satisfying couple sexual style, take personal responsibility for your sexuality and your growth as a unique, intimate team. You can be proud of yourselves for working together to address ED and maintain comfort and confidence with erections. In sharing emotional and sexual feelings and preferences, you increase understanding, empathy, and acceptance. This will provide the foundation for your couple sexual style that ensures both satisfaction and security.

10

Enjoying Sex and
Preventing Relapse

It took time, energy, and cooperation for you to confront ED and regain comfort and confidence with erections and intercourse. You cannot rest on your laurels; you need to devote time and energy to maintain a vital sexuality and prevent relapse. To expect that you will never have another experience where your erection is not sufficient for intercourse is unrealistic and sets you up for feelings of failure, a return to avoidance, and the blame-counterblame cycle. Positive, realistic expectations include accepting that arousal, erection, and intercourse are inherently variable. Whether once every ten times, once a month, or once a year, erectile problems will reoccur. This is a normal part of good-enough sex. The reality is that problems with desire, arousal, or orgasm are an occasional part of most couples' sexual experience. Especially important is to not panic and feel you are back to square one each time you experience an erectile problem. The key is to cooperate as an intimate team, accept the occasional episode of erectile problems as normal, treat it as a *lapse* (a single event which is not overly significant), shift to alternative scenarios, and commit to not allow it to become a *relapse* (a pattern perpetuated by anticipatory anxiety, hopelessness, and avoidance).

In this chapter, we'll help you develop an individualized, detailed relapse prevention plan. It is crucial that you decide how you'll respond when ED occurs rather than hope it will magically never happen again.

THE FOUNDATION OF RELAPSE PREVENTION

You can think about relapse prevention in terms of its cognitive, behavioral, and emotional aspects.

The Cognitive Foundation of Relapse Prevention

The crucial cognitive component is to accept that it is normal on occasion to not have an erection sufficient for intercourse. Treat these experiences as a normal variation, not a cue for anticipatory or performance anxiety. This allows you (and your partner) to think of the experience as a lapse not fear it will cause a relapse. A key to relapse prevention is shifting your focus from performance-oriented intercourse to involvement in the whole lovemaking process, affection through afterplay. Intercourse is a natural extension of intimacy, pleasuring, and eroticism, not a pass-fail test. Keep the perspective that you are sharing with your partner, not performing for her.

Think of your partner as your intimate friend whose pleasure and arousal feed yours rather than as a demanding critic for whom you must perform. Welcome her arousal rather than feeling intimidated. Enjoy both her arousal and your own. Enjoy your orgasm as well as her orgasm; orgasm need not occur in perfect sequence for sex to be satisfying.

Our concept of good-enough erectile function and good-enough couple sexuality is crucial for relapse prevention. You will feel genuinely satisfied with good-enough sex; you do not need to strive for perfect sex.

The Behavioral Foundation of Relapse Prevention

The most important behavioral strategy is to generalize the skills you learned systematically in the exercises and use them to maintain good-enough erectile function in unstructured, spontaneous sex. Integrate these techniques into your couple sexual style. If there is a break in your regular rhythm of sexual intercourse (if one of you has been traveling or has been ill), you may find it helpful to briefly return to using the techniques in a more structured way or to begin with an erotic, nonintercourse encounter.

Generally, you want sexual encounters that involve physical relaxation and a relaxed sexual pace; giving and receiving pleasure-oriented touching; blending sensual self-entrancement arousal and partner interaction arousal; openness to multiple stimulation during intercourse; transitioning to intercourse at a high level of arousal; varying intercourse positions and movements; moving to orgasm as a natural extension of the erotic flow; enjoying the orgasmic experience physically, emotionally, and relationally; and being an active participant in the afterplay phase. Be prepared to switch to erotic, nonintercourse sex or a cuddly, close scenario when intercourse is not possible.

It is important to maintain a regular rhythm of sexual experiences, with both people being involved and valuing their sexual relationship.

The Emotional Foundation of Relapse Prevention

An important relapse prevention approach is to value and reinforce your couple sexual style and to view each other as intimate friends. Positive feelings are the glue that binds you. Personal responsibility for sexuality, emotional sharing, and being an intimate team are ongoing parts of your life and relationship. Especially important is setting aside quality couple time when you share feelings—including feelings about your sexuality—empathically.

■ Nick and Amanda

Nick enjoyed what he thought of as "the sexy single life" until he met Amanda at thirty-five. When they married three years later, Amanda was thirty-four. Since they agreed they wanted two children, they started immediately and had two babies twenty months apart.

Nick was surprised to experience his first erectile problem at forty-three. The next two years were extremely frustrating for both Nick and Amanda. At first, Amanda told Nick this was normal and not to overreact, but Nick was not ready to accept any sexual difficulties. Nick and Amanda were an emotionally expressive couple, and ED led to intense fighting. Playful, erotic sex was replaced by high-intensity tears and anger. Nick had an impulsive affair to see if he was sexually functional with another woman (he got an erection, but lost it before intercourse), which contributed another layer of drama, guilt, and blame.

Amanda insisted they consult a marital therapist, who helped them confront and heal the emotional harm. She also helped Nick and Amanda realize that the emotionally expressive couple style no longer met their marital or family needs. They agreed to shift to a complementary marital style and recommit to a sexually monogamous marriage. Nick and Amanda naively hoped these relationship changes would automatically translate into better sex. However, the pattern of anticipatory and performance anxiety was well established, and the marital therapist suggested they work with a sex therapist.

Nick's ED was originally caused by his lack of knowledge about his body, stress and fatigue for both of them, and Nick's poor health habits. Once Nick became sensitized to erectile anxiety, several factors maintained his ED: the pattern of blaming, confusion, and ambivalence; Nick's anticipatory and performance anxiety; Amanda's low sexual desire; and her anxieties and inhibitions.

The sex therapist recommended a treatment plan to revitalize intimacy and sexuality. The first sexual exercise was to restart comfortable sensual touch. As often happens, Amanda's receptivity and responsiveness reminded Nick that sexuality can be a way to share pleasure rather than a demanding and failure-tinged sexual performance. Together, they worked through the steps of overcoming ED by focusing on relaxation, pleasure, and intimacy and accepting good-enough sex.

Amanda was more motivated than Nick to address relapse prevention issues. Nick was pleased with his erections and was afraid of jinxing it, but he too realized that he would have to work to maintain his progress. Amanda especially liked the idea of having a formal meeting every six months to discuss their relationship quality and intimacy and developing a new sexual scenario each year. Nick really enjoyed the boost in confidence he received from taking the Cialis his doctor prescribed, but he agreed with Amanda that their rekindled eroticism was a more powerful sexual stimulant than the drug. Amanda was fine with Nick taking Cialis as much or as little as he desired, but she wanted Nick to be open to spontaneous sexual encounters. Nick found it challenging to accept that it was okay to enjoy sensual or erotic scenarios when the sex did not flow to intercourse, but he realized that a pleasure orientation was healthier for both of them. Nick learned to stay erotically engaged with Amanda rather than retreating when he did not have an erection sufficient for intercourse. To help ensure that a lapse did not become a relapse, Nick decided that he would take Cialis the next time after a disappointing or dysfunctional sexual experience.

Even though they had heavy childcare responsibilities, two careers, and a busy life, Nick and Amanda set aside time to be an intimate couple. They expanded their idea of intimacy to include emotional closeness, affectionate and sensual touch, playful touching both in and out of the bedroom, enjoying a variety of pleasuring and erotic scenarios, and basking in afterplay. Nick and Amanda's new couple style valued erection and intercourse as well as emotional intimacy and eroticism.

RELAPSE PREVENTION STRATEGIES

The best relapse prevention strategy is for both you and your partner to commit to devoting the time and energy to maintain a high-quality intimate relationship. You do not need to devote hours a day; you can build intimacy through quick phone calls just to say hello, fifteen to thirty seconds of personal greeting when you come home, eye contact, kindnesses, listening, and empathy. Sexually, quality is based in maintaining a regular rhythm of affectionate, sensual, playful, erotic, and intercourse connection—whether three times a week or once every ten days—rather than regressing to the intercourse-or-nothing approach. But healthy sexuality is much more than frequency. A vital sexuality involves attending to physical health and healthy habits. Develop a relationship with your physician to ensure that an illness or medication side effect does not interfere with your sexual functioning. Be committed to enhancing your personal well-being and the well-being of your partner.

Here are ten relapse prevention strategies you can consider.

Strategy One: Hold Couple Meetings

Having regular times (for example, an hour or an afternoon each month) to discuss your intimate relationship is important for maintaining relational vitality and satisfaction. One advantage of working together to resolve ED or being in couple therapy is that you regularly engage in serious communication about your relationship. Continue to devote the time and energy to nurture and enhance your intimate relationship.

Strategy Two: Have a Formal Follow-Up Meeting

Planning a six-month follow-up (by yourselves or with a therapist) will help you remain committed and accountable to satisfying sex and prevent relapse by ensuring that you do not slip back into unhealthy sexual attitudes, behaviors, or feelings. The biggest trap is to treat ED and intimacy with benign neglect. If you don't pay attention, sex will regress to marginal quality and become infrequent.

Strategy Three: Have Pleasuring Sessions

Setting aside time for a pleasuring session (with a prohibition on orgasm) reinforces communication, sensuality, playfulness, and flexibility. This allows you to experiment and enjoy sensuality. This strategy combats relapse not just for ED but for other sexual problems, especially inhibited sexual desire.

Strategy Four: Calmly Accept Your Lapses as Simple Tests

In any change process, when you begin to achieve success, you will be tested. This is normal. When your new skills are challenged and you do a good-enough job of handling the test, you will be able to relax, settle in, and feel calmly confident. Your progress is for real, not a fluke. Your success becomes believable to both of you. You have learned the skills of sexual cooperation and intimacy.

As a couple, you will likely be tested a minimum of two or three times. The usual test is an experience of ED as severe as it ever was. You will have automatic thoughts of self-doubt: *This treatment approach didn't work. We're back at square one. I'm a sexual failure. We're going to return to the hurt, anger, and frustration.* While occasional negative thoughts are to be expected, you need to confront them and reaffirm that these fears are no longer valid.

When you are tested, what is important is that you pass the challenge together. You do this by handling the episode of ED with the cognitive, behavioral, emotional, and relationship skills you have learned and practiced. In other words, while you may not have an erection sufficient for intercourse, do not allow yourselves to relapse to handling it in the old dysfunctional way. You may elect to keep trying to get your erection by relaxing your PM and asking for sensual touch so you can relax your body. You are cooperating for pleasure. But do not invest more than five minutes trying to encourage an erection, because by then you'd probably be trying too hard and creating performance pressure.

Rather, accept that *this* encounter will not flow to intercourse, adapt your lovemaking, continue to pleasure and touch, and stay connected. Afterward, calmly discuss whether the lack of erection was simply a random event or whether there are some adjustments you will want to make together the next time you make love. These might include taking more time to relax your bodies, making love more slowly, focusing on pleasuring, using multiple stimulation, trying a new erotic scenario, taking a proerection medication, or having your partner initiate the transition to intercourse and guide intromission. Most important is to smile or shrug off the negative experience and make a date in the next three days when you have the time and energy for a sensuous, absorbing, erotic experience.

The better you pass the tests, the more assured your success will be. If you don't handle the testing well, it will take more practice. That is why it helps to consciously anticipate the tests so that you are not taken off guard. Remember, it is normal for up to 15 percent of sexual encounters to be dissatisfying or dysfunctional; do not overreact.

Strategy Five: Focus on Positive, Realistic Expectations

We hope that by now you've let go of your ideas about movie-type sex and erections that last for hours. If sexuality is to remain healthy and foster your intimate bond, you need to keep your expectations positive yet reasonable and to accept sexual variability and flexibility. Realistic, intimate sex will modulate with the events of your lives—the ease of vacation, the stress of parenting or careers, successes, illness. Adopt a broad-based approach to touching and eroticism. Remember that there are biological and psychological gender differences. Each couple needs to cooperatively find their way to accommodate each other's basic wants in realistic, respectful ways. Remember that there are multiple purposes for sex. Allow sexuality to meet a variety of individual and couple needs. Sometimes sex is a tension reducer; sometimes a way to share closeness; other times a short, passionate encounter, a way to heal an argument, a bridge to reduce emotional distance. It is a reality that sex is often better for one partner than the other. You can accept that sometimes sex will be better for her than for you.

Strategy Six: Schedule Intimate Couple Time

The importance of setting aside quality couple time cannot be emphasized enough. Nurture your relationship intimacy. For couples with children, it is especially important to set aside time together, whether a night out each week with cell phones turned off or a weekend without the children. Couples often report better sex on vacations, validating the importance of getting away, even for an hour or two. Couple time can include going for a walk, having a sexual date, going to dinner, having an intimate talk, or taking a half-hour nap.

Strategy Seven: Let Your Couple Sexual Style Develop over Time

There is not one right way to be sexual. Each couple develops their unique style of initiation, pleasuring, erotic scenarios and techniques, intercourse, and afterplay. The more flexible your couple sexual style and the more you accept the multiple functions of touching and sexuality, the greater your resistance to relapse. Develop a comfortable, functional, satisfying sexual style that meets both of your needs, flexibly adapts to the changes in your lives, and energizes your relationship.

Strategy Eight: Remember That Good-Enough Sex Varies

Be prepared to cope with disappointing or negative sexual experiences. The single most important technique in relapse prevention is to accept and not overreact to experiences that are mediocre or unsatisfying. Any couple can get along if everything goes well. The challenge is to accept disappointing experiences without panicking or blaming. Inhibited sexual desire, losing an erection, being fatigued, distractions you find hard to set aside, rapid ejaculation, female nonorgasmic response, a miscommunication about a sexual date: these happen to all couples. Take pride in having a resilient sexual style.

Strategy Nine: Saturate Each Other with Multidimensional Touch

Intimacy includes sexuality but is much more than sexual intercourse. You need a variety of intimate and erotic ways to connect, reconnect, and maintain connection. From time to time, remind yourselves of the type and proportion of touch you each enjoy, including affectionate touch, nongenital sensual touch, pleasurable genital touch, intercourse touch, and manual or oral erotic touch to orgasm. This gives you lots of tools to build bridges to sexual pleasure. The more ways you have to maintain intimate and sexual connection, the better you will avoid relapse.

Strategy Ten: Expand Your Sexual Repertoire

A flexible sexual and erotic repertoire is a major antidote to relapse. Sexuality that meets a range of needs, feelings, and situations will serve you well in maintaining erectile confidence and supporting your sexual and emotional gains. Couples who express intimacy through massage, holding hands, showering together, enjoying playful touch, engaging in semiclothed cuddling, and enjoying nude sensual touch have a flexible repertoire. You can build a robust sexual relationship by being open to "quickies," prolonged and varied erotic scenarios, various intercourse positions, multiple stimulation during intercourse, and planned as well as spontaneous sexual encounters.

CHOOSE YOUR RELAPSE PREVENTION STRATEGIES

With your partner, choose two to four relapse prevention strategies you believe could work for you. Then decide how to implement these strategies.

In movies and novels, once the problem is resolved, the couple lives happily ever after. In reality, your relationship and sexuality require time and at least periodic attention. We advocate an active relapse prevention program and, if sexuality gets off track, a problem-solving approach. Couples need to be able to deal with erectile problems and other sexual difficulties when they occur, but relapse *prevention* is easier and more effective. Why waste psychological energy dealing with a crisis when you can more efficiently and happily prevent the problem?

Rereading parts of this book from time to time is one way to keep yourselves well oriented amidst the distractions of life. Remember that realistic expectations are a key ingredient in sexual satisfaction. Accept that you will have occasional mediocre, disappointing, or failed sexual experiences. The more broadly based your sexual relationship, with emphasis on sharing desire, pleasure, eroticism, intercourse, and orgasm, the greater the likelihood you will cooperate as an intimate team, maintain your gains, and prevent relapse. This is good-enough sex.

You have come too far to relapse to ED and sexual performance anxiety. Confronting ED was a team effort. Maintaining and generalizing intimacy, sexual pleasure, arousal, and comfort with intercourse is likewise a team process. When people regress to ED, it is often the result of benign neglect. It is easy to procrastinate, be diverted by other things, fall into old habits, and let intimacy and sexuality slip down your list of priorities. Sexuality should not be the top priority in your relationship, but it should be a positive, integral component. You want to reinforce the positive feedback cycle of anticipation, pleasure, and a regular rhythm of sexual intercourse. Appreciate what you have overcome and what you have built together. Value enhanced intimacy, pleasure, and eroticism for you, your partner, and your relationship. Enjoy great sex together!

Choosing an Individual, Couple, or Sex Therapist

This is a self-help book, but it is not a do-it-yourself therapy book. Men and couples are often reluctant to consult a therapist, feeling that to do so is a sign of craziness, a confession of inadequacy, or an admission that your life and relationship are in dire straits. In reality, seeking professional help is a sign of psychological wisdom and strength. Entering individual, couple, or sex therapy means you realize there is a problem and you have made a commitment to resolve the issues and promote individual and couple growth.

The mental health field can be confusing. Couple and sex therapy are clinical subspecialties. They are offered by several groups of professionals, including psychologists, marital therapists, psychiatrists, social workers, nurses, and pastoral counselors. The professional background of the practitioner is less important than his or her competence in helping you deal with your ED and other specific problems.

Many people have health insurance that provides coverage for mental health, and thus can afford the services of a private practitioner. Those who do not have either the financial resources or insurance could consider a city or county mental health clinic, a university or medical school outpatient mental health clinic, or a family services center. Some clinics have a sliding fee scale (the fee is based on your ability to pay).

When choosing a therapist, be assertive in asking about credentials and areas of expertise. Ask the clinician what will be the focus of the therapy, how long therapy can be expected to last, and whether the emphasis is specifically on sexual problems or more generally on individual, communication, or relationship issues. Be especially diligent in asking about credentials such as university degrees and licensing. Be wary of people who call themselves personal counselors, sex counselors, or personal coaches. There are poorly qualified people—and some outright quacks—in any field.

One of the best ways to obtain a referral is to call a local professional organization such as a state psychological association, marriage and family therapy association, or mental health association. You can ask for a referral from a family physician, clergy or rabbi, or trusted friend. If you live near a university or medical school, call to find out what mental and sexual health services may be available.

For a sex therapy referral, contact the American Association of Sex Educators, Counselors, and Therapists (AASECT) through the Internet at www.aasect.org or write or call for a list of certified sex therapists in your area: P.O. Box 5488, Richmond, VA 23220; or call (804) 644-3288. Another resource is the Society for Sex Therapy and Research (SSTAR) at www.sstarnet.org.

For a marital therapist, check the Internet site for the American Association for Marriage and Family Therapy (AAMFT) at www.therapistlocator.net. The Association for the Advancement of Behavior Therapy (AABT) at www.aabt.com has resources for locating individual and couple therapists.

Feel free to talk with two or three therapists before deciding on one with whom to work. Be aware of your level of comfort with the therapist, degree of rapport, whether the therapist has special skill working with couples, and whether the therapist's assessment of the problem and approach to treatment makes sense to you.

Once you begin, give therapy a chance to be helpful. There are few miracle cures. Change requires commitment and is a gradual and often difficult process. Although some people benefit from short-term therapy (fewer than ten sessions), most find the therapeutic process will require four months or longer. The role of the therapist is that of a consultant rather than a decision maker. Therapy requires effort, both in the sessions and at home. Therapy helps to change attitudes, feelings, and behavior. Although it takes courage to seek professional help, therapy can be a tremendous help in evaluating and changing individual, relational, and sexual problems.

Resources

SUGGESTED READING ON MALE SEXUALITY

Joannides, Paul. 1999. *The Guide to Getting It On.* West Hollywood, Calif.: The Goofy Foot Press.

McCarthy, Barry, and Emily McCarthy. 1998. *Male Sexual Awareness.* New York: Carroll and Graf.

Milsten, Richard, and Julian Slowinski. 1999. *The Sexual Male: Problems and Solutions.* New York: W.W. Norton & Company.

Pryor, Jon L. and Stacy Glass. 2000. *It's in the Male: Everyone's Guide to Men's Health.* Minneapolis: Appladay Press.

Zilbergeld, Bernie. 1999. *The New Male Sexuality.* New York: Bantam Books.

SUGGESTED READING ON FEMALE SEXUALITY

Ellison, Carol. 2001. *Women's Sexualities.* Oakland, Calif.: New Harbinger Publications.

Foley, Sallie, Sally Kope, and Dennis Sugrue. 2002. *Sex Matters for Women: A Complete Guide to Taking Care of Your Sexual Self.* New York: Guilford Publications.

Goodwin, Aurelie, and Marc Agronin. 1997. *A Woman's Guide to Overcoming Sexual Fear and Pain.* Oakland, Calif.: New Harbinger Publications.

Heiman, Julian, and Joseph LoPiccolo. 1988. *Becoming Orgasmic: Women's Guide to Sexual Fulfillment.* New York: Prentice-Hall.

Leiblum, Sandra, and Judith Sachs. 2002. *Getting the Sex You Want: A Woman's Guide to Becoming Proud, Passionate, and Pleased in Bed.* New York: Crown Publishers.

SUGGESTED READING ON COUPLE SEXUALITY

Holstein, Lana. 2002. *How to Have Magnificent Sex: The Seven Dimensions of a Vital Sexual Connection*. New York: Harmony Books.

McCarthy, Barry, and Emily McCarthy. 1998. *Couple Sexual Awareness*. New York: Carroll and Graf.

McCarthy, Barry, and Emily McCarthy. 2002. *Sexual Awareness: Couple Sexuality for the Twenty-First Century*. New York: Carroll and Graf.

Schnarch, David. 1997. *Passionate Marriage: Sex, Love and Intimacy in Emotionally Committed Relationships*. New York: W.W. Norton.

OTHER NOTABLE SEXUALITY READINGS

Butler, Robert, and Myrna Lewis. 2002. *The New Love and Sex after Sixty*. New York: Ballantine.

Maltz, Wendy. 2001. *The Sexual Healing Journey*. New York: HarperCollins.

McCarthy, Barry, and Emily McCarthy. 2003. *Rekindling Desire*. New York: Brunner/Routledge.

Metz, Michael, and Barry McCarthy. 2003. *Coping with Premature Ejaculation: Overcome PE, Please Your Partner, and Have Great Sex*. Oakland, Calif.: New Harbinger Publications.

Michael, Robert, John Gagnon, Edward Laumann, and Gina Kolata. 1994. *Sex in America: A Definitive Survey*. New York: Little, Brown, and Company.

Weiner-Davis, Michelle. 2003. *The Sex-Starved Marriage*. New York: Simon and Schuster.

Zoldbrod, Aline. *Sex Smart*. 1998. Oakland, Calif.: New Harbinger Publications.

SUGGESTED READING ON RELATIONSHIP SATISFACTION

Chapman, Gary. 1995. *The Five Love Languages: How to Express Heartfelt Commitment to Your Mate*. Chicago: Northfield Publishing.

Doherty, William. 2001. *Take Back Your Marriage*. New York: Guilford Press.

Gottman, John. 1999. *The Seven Principles for Making Marriage Work.* New York: Crown Publishing.

Markman, Howard, Scott Stanley, and Susan L. Blumberg. 2001. *Fighting for Your Marriage: Positive Steps for Preventing Divorce and Preserving a Lasting Love.* San Francisco: Jossey-Bass Publishers.

McCarthy, Barry, and Emily McCarthy. 2004. *Getting It Right the First Time: Creating a Healthy Marriage.* New York: Brunner/Routledge.

SUGGESTED READING AND RESOURCES FOR MENTAL HEALTH

Burns, David. 1989. *The Feeling Good Handbook.* New York: Penguin Books.

Bourne, Edmund. 2001. *The Anxiety and Phobia Workbook.* Third edition. Oakland, Calif.: New Harbinger Publications.

Obsessive-Compulsive Foundation
www.ocfoundation.org

National Institutes of Mental Health (NIMH)
Home page: www.nimh.nih.gov
Anxiety: www.nimh.nih.gov/anxiety/anxietymenu.cfm
Depression: www.nimh.nih.gov/publicat/depressionmenu.cfm

CHEMICAL DEPENDENCY RESOURCES

The Hazelden Foundation
www.hazelden.org
(800) 328-9000, fax (651) 213-4590
15251 Pleasant Valley Road, Box 196, Center City, MN 55012

SMOKING CESSATION

Mayo Clinic Nicotine Dependence Center
www.mayoclinic.org/ndc-rst

United States Surgeon General, tobacco cessation information
www.surgeongeneral.gov/tobacco

RESOURCES FOR HEALTH CONCERNS

Medline Plus, a service of the U.S. National Library and the National
  Institutes of Health
  www.medlineplus.gov

PROFESSIONAL ASSOCIATIONS

American Association for Marriage and Family Therapy (AAMFT)
  www.therapistlocator.net
American Association of Sex Educators, Counselors, and Therapists
  (AASECT)
  P.O. Box 5488, Richmond, VA 23220-0488
  (804) 644-3288
  www.aasect.org
Association for the Advancement of Behavioral Therapy (AABT)
  305 Seventh Avenue, New York, NY 10001-6008
  (212) 647-1890
  www.aabt.org
Sex Information and Education Council of the United States (SIECUS)
  130 West 42nd Street, Suite 350, New York, NY 10036
  (212) 819-7990, fax (212) 819-9776
  www.seicus.org
Society for Sex Therapy and Research (SSTAR)
  www.sstarnet.org
Society for Scientific Study of Sexuality (SSSS): David Fleming, Execu-
  tive Director.
  P.O. Box 416, Allentown, PA 18105-0416
  (610) 530-2483
  www.sexscience.org

SEX "TOYS," BOOKS, AND VIDEOS

Good Vibrations Mail Order
  938 Howard Sreet, Suite 101, San Francisco, CA 94110.
  (800) 289-8423, fax (415) 974-8990
  www.goodvibes.com

VIDEOTAPES: SEXUAL ENRICHMENT

Holstein, Lana. 2001. *Magnificent Lovemaking.* 79 min. Canyon Ranch Bookstore, Tucson, AZ 85750. (520) 749-9000, extension 4380.

Perry, Michael, and Goedele Liekens. 1991. *Sex: A Lifelong Pleasure* series. Sinclair Intimacy Institute, P.O. Box 8865, Chapel Hill, NC 27515. (800) 955-0888, fax (800) 794-3318
www.intimacyinstitute.com or www.bettersex.com.

Sommers, Frank. 1992. *The Great Sex Video Series.* 75 min. Distributor: Pathway Productions, Inc., 360 Bloor Street West, Suite 407A, Toronto M5S 1X1 CANADA. (416) 922-4506, fax (416) 922-7512. E-mail: how2video@aol.com.

Stubbs, Kenneth Ray. 1994. *Erotic Massage.* 58 min. Secret Garden, P.O. Box 67, Larkspur, CA 94977.

The Couples Guide to Great Sex Over 40, volumes 1 and 2. 1995. Sinclair Intimacy Institute, P.O. Box 8865, Chapel Hill, NC 27515. (800) 955-0888, fax (800) 794-3318.
www.intimacyinstitute.com or www.bettersex.com

References

Amen, D. G. 1998. *Change Your Brain, Change Your Life.* New York: Three Rivers Press.

Bailey, J., and R. C. Pillard. 1995. Genetics of human sexual orientation. *Annual Review of Sex Research* 6:126–50.

Basson, R. 2001. Using a different model for female sexual response to address women's problematic low sexual desire. *Journal of Sex and Marital Therapy* 27:395–403.

Cabaj, R. P., and T. S. Stein, eds. 1996. *Textbook of Homosexuality and Mental Health.* Arlington, Va.: American Psychiatric Publishing, Inc.

Cocores, J., and M. Gold. 1989. Substance abuse and sexual dysfunction. *Medical Aspects of Human Sexuality* February: 22–31.

Cummins, T., and S. Miller. 2003. The effects of drug abuse on sexual functioning. In *Handbook of Clinical Sexuality for Mental Health Professionals*, edited by S. Levine, C. Risen, and S. Althof. New York: Brunner/Routledge.

Diego, M. A., T. Field, M. Hernandez-Reif, J. A. Shaw, E. M. Rothe, D. Castellanos, and L. Mesner. 2002. Aggressive adolescents benefit from massage therapy. *Adolescence* 37(147):597–607.

Fagan, P. 2002. Psychogenic impotency in relatively young men. In *Handbook of Clinical Sexuality*, edited by S. Levine, C. Risen, and S. Althof. New York: Brunner/Routledge.

Feldman, H., I. Goldstein, D. Hatzichristou, R. Krane, and J. McKinlay. 1994. Impotence and its medical and psychosocial correlates: Results of the Massachusetts Male Aging Study. *Journal of Urology* 151:54–61.

Frank, E., C. Anderson, and D. Rubenstein. 1978. Frequency of sexual dysfunction in "normal" couples. *New England Journal of Medicine* 229(3):111–15.

Jamison, P., and P. Gebhard. 1988. Penis size increase between flaccid and erect states: An analysis of the Kinsey data. *Journal of Sex Research* 24:177– 83.

Kaplan, H. S. 1974. *The New Sex Therapy*. New York: Brunner/Mazel.

Laumann, E., J. Gagnon, R. Michael, and S. Michaels. 1994. *The Social Organization of Sexuality: Sexual Practices in the United States*. Chicago: University of Chicago Press.

Loudon, J. B. 1998. Potential confusion between erectile dysfunction and premature ejaculation: An evaluation of men presenting with erectile difficulty at a sex therapy clinic. *Sexual and Marital Therapy* 13(4): 397–401.

Masters, W. H., and V. E. Johnson. 1966. *Human Sexual Response*. Boston: Little, Brown, and Company.

———. 1970. *Human Sexual Inadequacy*. Boston: Little, Brown, and Company.

Michael, R., J. Gagnon, E. Laumann, and G. Kolata. 1994. *Sex in America: A Definitive Survey*. New York: Little, Brown, and Company.

Moore, T. M., J. L. Strauss, S. Herman, and C. F. Donatucci. 2003. Erectile dysfunction in early, middle, and late adulthood: Symptom patterns and psychosocial correlates. *Journal of Sex and Marital Therapy* 29(5):381–99.

Mosher, D. L. 1980. Three psychological dimensions of depth of involvement in human sexual response. *Journal of Sex Research* 16(1):1–42.

Olson, M., and N. Sneed. 1995. Anxiety and therapeutic touch. *Issues in Mental Health Nursing* 16(2):97–108.

Pillard, R. C., and J. M. Bailey. 1995. A biologic perspective on sexual orientation. *Psychiatric Clinics of North America* 18(1):71–84.

Robinson, L. 1996. The effects of therapeutic touch on the grief experience. *Dissertation Abstracts International: Section B: The Sciences & Engineering* 56(11-B):6039.

Schatzberg, A. F., and C. B. Nemeroff. 2004. *Textbook of Psychopharmacology*. 3rd ed. Arlington, Va.: American Psychiatric Publishing, Inc.

Segraves, R. T., and R. Balon. 2003. *Sexual Pharmacology: Fast Facts*. New York: W. W. Norton.

Sidi, A., P. K. Reddy, and K. K. Chen. 1988. Patient acceptance of and satisfaction with vasoactive intracavernous pharmacotherapy for impotence. *Journal of Urology* 140:293–97.

Weeks, G., and N. Gambescia. 2000. *Erectile Dysfunction*. New York: W. W. Norton.

Zoldbrod, A. 1993. *Men, Women, and Infertility*. New York: W. W. Norton.

WE WANT YOUR CANDID FEEDBACK:

We are very interested in your response to our book and welcome your feedback. For example:

- Why did you buy our book?

- What has been helpful to you?

- What about our approach do you most like?

- What do you wish we had addressed more fully?

Please send an e-mail or letter with your comments, requests, or ideas to:

CopingWithED@aol.com

Or:

Michael E. Metz, Ph.D.
Meta Associates
Baker Court, Suite 440
821 Raymond Avenue
St. Paul, MN 55114

Barry W. McCarthy, Ph.D.
Washington Psychological Center
4201 Connecticut Avenue, N.W.
Suite 602
Washington, DC 20008

WE WELCOME YOUR REQUESTS:

We also welcome requests to present workshops, training sessions, and lectures about ED, sexual health, and marital and sexual wellness.

Thank you very much. Michael Metz and Barry McCarthy.

Michael E. Metz, Ph.D., works in the Twin Cities of Minneapolis and St. Paul, Minnesota and is one of the country's leading sexologists in the area of healthy male and couple sexuality. He is a major spokesperson for a comprehensive, integrated biopsychosocial approach to addressing and resolving sexual problems. After twelve years on the faculty of the University of Minnesota Medical School, he currently works in private practice with Meta Associates as a psychologist, marital therapist, and sex therapist treating individuals and couples, and is affiliated with the University of Minnesota's Department of Family Social Science. He has published more than forty-five professional articles and conducted numerous workshops and talks on marital and sex therapy. He is the author of the *Styles of Conflict Inventory (SCI)*, a clinical assessment instrument to evaluate the conflict patterns in relationships; and together with Dr. McCarthy, *Coping with Premature Ejaculation*

Barry W. McCarthy, Ph.D., is a clinical psychologist with a subspecialty in marriage and sex therapy practicing at the Washington Psychological Center in Washington, DC. He is professor of psychology at American University, where he teaches an undergraduate human sexual behavior course. Barry, with his wife Emily, has written seven well-respected books, the most recent being *Rekindling Desire: A Step By Step Program to Help Low-Sex and No-Sex Marriages, Sexual Awareness: Couple Sexuality for the Twenty-First Century*, and *Getting It Right the First Time: Creating a Healthy Marriage*. He is also the author with Dr. Metz of *Coping with Premature Ejaculation*. In addition, he has published over fifty-five professional articles, and fourteen book chapters, and has presented over one hundred fifty highly acclaimed workshops nationally and internationally.

Some Other
New Harbinger Titles

Eating Mindfully, Item 3503, $13.95

Living with RSDS, Item 3554 $16.95

The Ten Hidden Barriers to Weight Loss, Item 3244 $11.95

The Sjogren's Syndrome Survival Guide, Item 3562 $15.95

Stop Feeling Tired, Item 3139 $14.95

Responsible Drinking, Item 2949 $18.95

The Mitral Valve Prolapse/Dysautonomia Survival Guide, Item 3031 $14.95

Stop Worrying Abour Your Health, Item 285X $14.95

The Vulvodynia Survival Guide, Item 2914 $15.95

The Multifidus Back Pain Solution, Item 2787 $12.95

Move Your Body, Tone Your Mood, Item 2752 $17.95

The Chronic Illness Workbook, Item 2647 $16.95

Coping with Crohn's Disease, Item 2655 $15.95

The Woman's Book of Sleep, Item 2493 $14.95

The Trigger Point Therapy Workbook, Item 2507 $19.95

Fibromyalgia and Chronic Myofascial Pain Syndrome, second edition, Item 2388 $19.95

Kill the Craving, Item 237X $18.95

Rosacea, Item 2248 $13.95

Thinking Pregnant, Item 2302 $13.95

Shy Bladder Syndrome, Item 2272 $13.95

Help for Hairpullers, Item 2329 $13.95

Coping with Chronic Fatigue Syndrome, Item 0199 $13.95

Call **toll free, 1-800-748-6273,** or log on to our online bookstore at **www.newharbinger.com** to order. Have your Visa or Mastercard number ready. Or send a check for the titles you want to New Harbinger Publications, Inc., 5674 Shattuck Ave., Oakland, CA 94609. Include $4.50 for the first book and 75¢ for each additional book, to cover shipping and handling. (California residents please include appropriate sales tax.) Allow two to five weeks for delivery.

Prices subject to change without notice.